# SOCIAL DEVELOPMENT

to the memory of H.B.

**Studies in Developmental Paediatrics**
Series Editor Margaret Pollak

Volume 4

# SOCIAL DEVELOPMENT

## Ruth Blunden

Senior Psychologist
Sir Wilfrid Sheldon Children's Centre
King's College Hospital Medical School
London

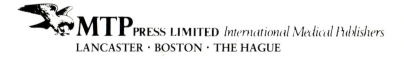
**MTP**PRESS LIMITED *International Medical Publishers*
LANCASTER · BOSTON · THE HAGUE

Published in the UK and Europe by
MTP Press Limited
Falcon House
Lancaster, England

**British Library Cataloguing in Publication Data**
Blunden, Ruth
  Social development.—(Studies in developmental
  paediatrics; v. 4)
  1. Socialization
  I. Title
  303.3'2      HQ783
  ISBN  0-85200-304-8

Published in the USA by
MTP Press
A division of Kluwer Boston
190 Old Derby Street
Hingham, MA 02043, USA

**Library of Congress Cataloging in Publication Data**
Blunden, Ruth.
  Social development.

  (Studies in developmental paediatrics; v. 4)
  Includes bibliographical references and index.
  1. Socialization.   2. Child development.
  I. Title.  II. Series. [DNLM: 1. Child development.
  2. Socialization. WS 105.5.S6 B658s]
  HQ783.B56      303.3'2  /  81-20862
  ISBN  0-85200-304-8  /  AACR2

Printed in Great Britain by
Butler & Tanner Ltd, Frome and London

# CONTENTS

**Studies in Developmental Paediatrics**

*Other books in the series include:*

Language Development and Assessment – Joan Reynell

The Development of Hearing – Sybil Yeates

The Development of Vision – P. A. Gardiner

Neuromuscular Development – P. Robson

Adaptive Development – Margaret Pollak

# SERIES EDITOR'S NOTE

Adequate social development is a necessity for all children in order that they may live and interact happily and successfully with their families, friends and society.

If adequate social development is important for all children, nowhere is it more essential than for the handicapped. Often, by concentrating upon the fulfilment of potential in social skills, the severely handicapped can become more acceptable to society and thus live within it rather than suffer segregation and isolation.

Although subject – as are all parameters of development – to the basic rules of development, social development is somewhat different to the other parameters for several reasons:

It is often not seen in isolation but superimposed upon other aspects of behaviour. It is seen in the home, nursery, school and street.

It is subject, in a marked degree, to environmental and cultural attitudes and is thus affected by child rearing practices, social class and ethnic group.

Wide swings and 'ups' and 'downs' can be expected in individual children so that wide variations are allowable. These are, in part, due to the emotional content of social behaviour – mood and stress both affecting performance.

Ruth Blunden's excellent book brings these – and many other – points out with telling description and, furthermore, she backs up her views with the findings of many research studies.

She reminds us that social development begins at birth and describes the aspects and problems of different ages through to adolescence. We need to know what is the current thinking about the effect upon children of many aspects of modern living – for example television and the media – yet such knowledge is not easy to find.

I believe that the chapters on adolescence and treatment will prove to be particularly helpful.

But, perhaps most helpful of all, by accepting that early experiences, whilst important, are not irreversible, Ruth Blunden gives those of us engaged in continuing care hope and optimism and the encouragement to attempt change.

I hope this volume will be available in Child Guidance clinics as well as in paediatric, community and family doctor consulting rooms.

Margaret Pollak
Consultant Paediatrician to the Sir Wilfrid Sheldon
    Assessment Centre
Senior Lecturer in Developmental, Social and Educational
    Paediatrics
King's College Hospital
London SE5

# INTRODUCTION

This book tries to trace the course of social development in the child from birth to maturity. It assumes that the neonate comes into the world with the endowment and the need to contact others, to attach itself to the surrounding humans and by this very endowment enforces these humans to attach themselves to it. The book follows the main vicissitudes in this process and describes in short outlines some of the disturbing manifestations of failure at different ages in the smooth progress of socialization – the process by which the child adapts to the requirements of the social group of which he is a member.

In accordance with recent studies the book stresses the influence on social development of the wider environment. It is no longer believed that the quality of the early mother–child relationship exclusively determines all later development.

The book also surveys the present state of assessment and treatment methods and tries to indicate where short intervention by the developmental paediatrician might be sufficient and where more long-term intensive treatment by specialists would be needed. The author agrees with A. M. and A. D. B. Clarke (1976) that early experiences, though powerful, are not irreversible, and that with changes in environmental circumstances, and with understanding of the main causal factors for the deviance, the effect of adverse early events may be modified and development towards normal social progress may to some extent be restored.

# ACKNOWLEDGEMENTS

This book relies on evidence that has been developed and interpreted during the last decade by English and American psychologists, psychiatrists and paediatricians. They are extensively quoted and the length of the reference list reflects the diversity of the field.

The insights gained by the reseachers and their interpreters has been confirmed or modified by my own observations during long years of professional contact with sick and healthy infants, deprived and disturbed toddlers and schoolchildren, emotionally vulnerable young adolescents, and with the families of these children.

I was given the opportunity to watch the children during my years as staff member in the psychiatric and paediatric departments of two teaching hospitals in London, the Charing Cross Hospital and the King's Cross Hospital. I am indebted to the consultants, particularly Professor C. E. Stroud, Professor of Child Health at King's College, to Dr Margaret Pollak, Director of the Sir Wilfrid Sheldon Children's Centre, Consultant Paediatrician and Senior Lecturer in Developmental, Educational and Social Paediatrics, King's College Hospital Medical School, to Dr Lorna Wheelan, Consultant Psychiatrist and Director of the Clinic of Child and Family Therapy, Belgrave Hospital for Children, and also to Drs J. Randell and G. Oppenheim, consultant psychiatrists at Charing Cross Hospital, whose young adolescents I was permitted to see.

I also owe thanks to the registrars and other professionals at Charing Cross and King's Cross with whom I discussed cases and learned about therapeutic methods and problems. My most fervent thanks, of course, go to the children themselves with their fascinating and variable individualities, their family entanglements and their gratifying responsiveness to a stranger.

This book could not have been written without the support of my sister, Katrina de Hirsch, Special Consultant in Psychiatry at Columbia University and former Director of the Pediatric Language Disorder Clinic at Columbia Presbyterian Medical Center, New York City. In long and fervent discussions and controversies about the children's problems, I profited from her rich experience with children from entirely different backgrounds from those I saw in London. I cannot say how much I owe to her encouragement, criticism and advice.

# Chapter 1

---

# COMMUNICATING WITH THE INFANT

---

## (A) THE BABY'S SOCIAL COMPETENCE

'We are eavesdropping on a fundamental process of human socialisation of whose very existence developmental psychologists have previously been unaware' wrote Schaffer in 1971, expressing the intense astonishment experienced by paediatricians and psychologists in the early seventies. Almost suddenly, by new methods of infant observation, it became possible to watch in minute detail infants asleep and awake in their cots, and mothers and infants playing and talking together in the hospital or at home. It was then recognized that the human infant is not only born with a far greater range of cognitive skills than anyone had known, not only with individual characteristics sharply distinguishing one infant from another, but is also – and more astonishingly – 'pre-programmed with some kind of sensitivity towards reciprocal interaction. Within days or mere hours after birth it is embarked upon the never ending program of social intercommunication with other human beings' (Newson 1979).

In 1971 Schaffer began his book *The Growth of Sociability* with the words: 'At birth the infant is essentially an a-social being.' The fact, however, is, that infants are born into a social world and at once begin to interact with this world. After the intense growth of research about human social development, which has occurred since then, I doubt whether Schaffer would again stress that the neonate is asocial, particularly since we owe to him a good deal of the insights we have since acquired. If social competence is defined as 'the ability to elicit the co-operation of others' (Ainsworth 1974) and 'central to this social competence is effective communication, then the neonate's first signalling behaviour, i.e. his crying is present on the first day and exerts a measure of control over others' (his mother). The growth of this social competence is rapid and before the first 6 months of life the infant's social capabilities are, indeed, formidable. He is fully ready to engage in the first phase of learning and interacting with the human world (Stern 1977).

## (B) TECHNIQUES OF INFANT OBSERVATION

In 1961, the Fantz apparatus – a contraption placed over the cot where, by a clever arrangement of mirrors, it becomes possible to see which sort of visual display the baby is most interested in – had already clearly shown that the infant prefers designs resembling the human face to all others. Just as the baby is selectively attuned to the human voice (the crying neonate is quietened by sounds within the speech range) it comes into the world with a clear preference for visual patterns having the main features of the human face. At the age of 6 days a disc with an oval design and prominent dots as eyes, showing the light–dark contrast seen in human faces, is clearly more attractive to the infant than any other patterns and this design will soon elicit smiles (Figure 1). (The preference is entirely indiscriminate and four eye spots are even more attractive than two – similar to the seagulls which retrieve artificial eggs rather than their own eggs, provided the artificial eggs are bigger but otherwise resemble the real eggs.)

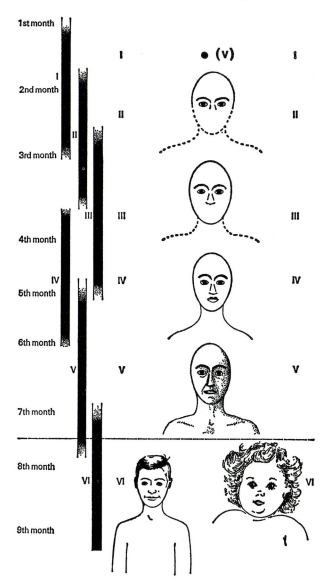

Figure 1   Necessary and sufficient conditions for evoking smiling in infants up to the ninth month [from Schaffer (1971)]

In the Fantz apparatus the infant is observed lying in the cot on his back; however, babies behave very differently when picked up and, face to face with mother or caretaker, will watch the world from the upright position. In fact, a lying infant is probably always half asleep. Lying for hours on end in a cot, day by day, as was once usual in institutions, is undoubtedly detrimental to the baby's development (Dennis and Najaran 1957). The new techniques, to which we owe our recent insights, take account of the fact that the baby must and will be part of things.

Long before the baby can sit up on his own, or hold his head steadily upright, he is propped up in a specially designed cushion with head support and mother plays with the infant. By an arrangement of mirrors, which shows both partners' faces, baby and mother are videotaped or filmed simultaneously while playing together. The films have delicate timers attached to them and can be played

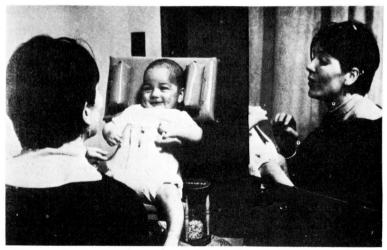

Figure 2  Examples of mother–infant play [reproduced from *Studies in Mother–Infant Interaction* (ed. Schaffer, H. R., 1977), pp. 236 and 244–5, copyright by Academic Press Inc. (London) Ltd., by kind permission of the publishers and Dr C. Trevarthen]

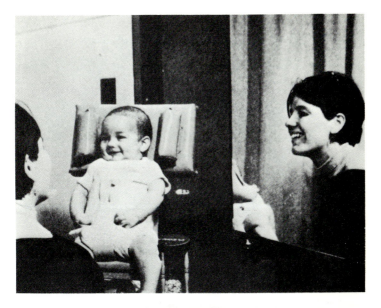

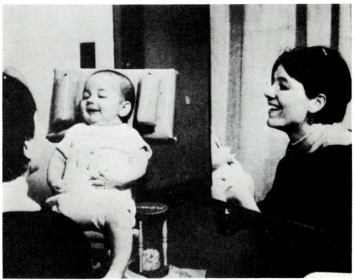

Figure 2 (continued)

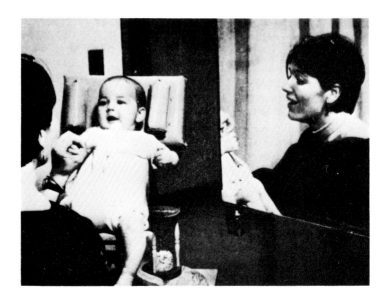

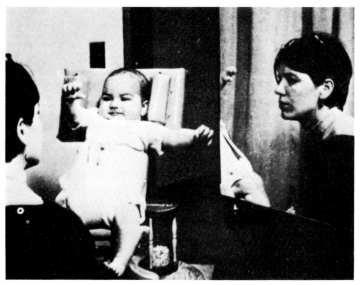

Figure 2 (continued)

back in slow motion and scrutinized frame by frame (by tenths of seconds). Sophisticated techniques of analysis of soundtracks have been added and observations are being made within the first hours after delivery in hospital, or in the early days at home. They have utterly demolished the idea of the newborn infant being only a bundle of sensations, utterly passive, 'assailed' – in James's (1890) famous words – 'by eyes, ears, nose, skin and entrails all at once, feeling it all as one blooming buzzing confusion'. In 1928 Watson, the father of behaviourism, had said 'the human being at birth is a lowly piece of unformed protoplasm ready to be shaped by any family in whose care it is placed'; this is now known to be utterly untrue (Figure 2).

## (C) SOCIAL SIGNALLING DEVICES

Evidence has now accumulated which shows that the human being is hugely precocious, socially. It is biologically primed and pretuned to communicate with other humans long before it shares a linguistic code with them.

Microanalysis of videotapes shows that the infant, less than 2 months old, may not only express communicative messages by its facial movements, but can also perceive and locate communicative acts of partners. The infant prefers more than any other object the visual presentation of upright full views of face-like shapes, prefers raised eyebrows, movements of mouth and cheek indicating smiles, and auditory stimuli with the pitch and articulation of the human voice. This is so even if these features are presented mechanically and by machines. However, the infant's response is more intense and immediate when these features are combined as patterns, such as those that occur only when people are willing to communicate with the infant.

The baby has an astonishingly mature facial musculature with which it can – at first only by reflex – simulate expres-

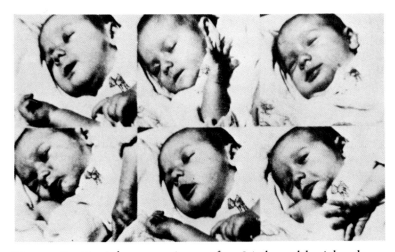

Figure 3    Facial expressions of a 24-day-old girl asleep [reproduced from *Before Speech* (ed. Bullowa, M., 1979), p. 326, Cambridge University Press, by kind permission of the publishers and Dr C. Trevarthen]

sions of emotion, even in the first days of life, before the expressions become meaningful (Figure 3). By 5-8 weeks these facial expressions exert a powerful influence over the adults caring for the infant. Mothers and nurses react emotionally to these 'signalling devices' and the fact that the baby enforces in this way emotional responses from the adult is important. The infant's expressions are not learned from the adult. Interaction tapes show that it is the adult who mimics the baby rather than the baby who mimics the adult.

## (D)  THE PRE-SPEECH DIALOGUE

Infants' responses to people are totally different from their responses to objects: psychologists had believed that in the field of parent-infant relations the infant's behaviour was a function of his parents; now we know that at least some parental behaviours are directly instigated by those of their children. Brazelton (1973), who constructed a test for the newborn, predictive of his future central nervous system organization, says 'the newborn comes equipped with a series of complex behaviours for eliciting the appropriate nurturing behaviour responses from the adults around him'.

Up to 6 months of age a child may appear 'blind' to even brightly coloured stationary objects when they are clearly within his field of vision. For instance, a red cube on a black table-top may be stared at, but it is reached for only when special attention is drawn to it by jiggling, rattling, etc. On the other hand, attention is rapidly caught by mobile noise-emitting devices, such as humans are. Moreover, humans tend to respond to the infant. When the infant is given an interesting object to look at, the eyes narrow, body posture becomes tense and fingers and arms are orientated towards the object in an incipient pointing gesture. Attention is then followed by an abrupt turning away. With people, on the other hand, there is a repeated cycle – the eyes widen instead of narrowing, the face is mobile, smiling is common, the body is relaxed and there is a cycle which goes from greeting to disengagement to repeated greeting and disengagement in a smooth rhythm, almost like a dance. It is clear that even at 2–3 months the baby can distinguish animate from inanimate objects.

Adults make the assumption that the infant is attempting some form of meaningful dialogue – the infant emits signs and the care-giver endows the signs with social significance and thus a shared meaning gradually begins to take place.

Trevarthen (1979) says that his observations have led him to accept the idea 'that human beings are equipped at birth with a mechanism which is sensitive to persons and expresses itself as a person does' adding that 'obviously such a mechanism must be formulated largely within the brain before birth without benefit of imitation and training'. He says that cross-cultural studies give evidence of an 'innate pan-human vocabulary' of emotional signs.

The mechanism of language already functions in early infancy: mothers, when talking to their infants, do this by using rhythmic sounds with exaggerated facial displays to retain the infants' attention. The infant in turn synchronizes its gestures and vocalizations, his gurgles and grunts and babbles, in the same rhythm – there is a game of turn-taking, revealing an astonishing innate time sense of the baby, of which we formerly had no idea. This enables the infant to engage in 'conversations' before it begins to speak. Exact experimental monitoring of the vocal exchanges between mothers and infants have shown that overlap is rare. Baby vocalizes when mother pauses, and mother coos or sings or talks when baby pauses.

Interestingly, even when the infant's talk carries no linguistic information there is an interaction which shares the characteristics of verbal conversation; clearly, in adult conversation one partner also waits for the other to give a signal for him to speak, since no one can speak and listen at the same time.

## (E) EXPERIMENTAL MANIPULATION OF COMMUNICATION

But what happens when this give and take, elicitation and response, goes wrong? There are by now many studies concerned with the abnormal as well as the normal mother–infant interaction, some of them experimentally induced: Bower, in Edinburgh, has had mothers looking at their infants through a soundproof window and loudspeakers arranged so as to make her voice appear to come from either her mouth or from a different part of the room, When mother's voice came from a different direction children became distressed, indicating expectancy which was violated and causing upset even in these early days.

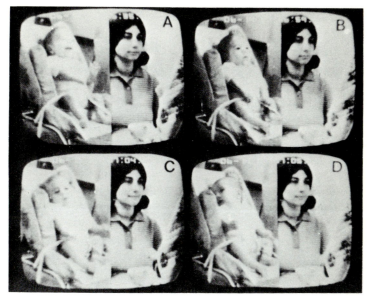

Figure 4    Mother still-faced, baby watching [reproduced from *Before Speech* (ed. Bullowa, M., 1979), p. 365, Cambridge University Press, by kind permission]

When adults are unresponsive, avoiding or aggressive, 2-month-old infants show tension and distress by yawning, grimacing, frowning, gaze avoidance and even startle movements.

If a mother is made to freeze her expression in the middle of a happy communicative exchange – which they find very hard to do – the infant may stare at her face with expression of appeal or solicitation (Figure 4). At 10 weeks it may briefly smile, then run through its repertoire of facial expressions and limb movements, attempting to initiate normal happy interaction. Finally it will avert its gaze entirely.

On the other hand, if mothers were told to slow down their speech, which is naturally already much slower than normal speech, and much more simple and repetitive, babies at first seem perplexed: they watch mother for a bit but then they return happily to the exchange, even increasing it and enjoying the new game of slowed-up 'conversation' (Tronick *et al.* 1979). In a motor car with mother driving, showing only her profile to the baby, the baby seldom smiles but may make cooing, calling vocalizations or even cry (but the cry seems faked), evidence for the sensitivity of the child to the partner's manner of communication.

The sensitivity of mother to the baby's signalling devices has become a central issue in research: the baby's crying clearly has no intentional context until 8-9 months of life – i.e. baby does not *intend* by his cry to get mother's attention – nevertheless, mother's responsiveness to baby's cry, right from the start, promotes the infant's communication and hence his social competence. Ainsworth *et al.*'s (1974) research – which tabulated both the frequency and duration of the infant's crying as well as the frequency of mother's ignoring the cry and the lapse of time before her response – showed that mother's responsiveness does not exert any influence on the infant's 'signalling device' within the first 3 months of life (in contrast to learning theory, which would predict extinction of the crying by lack of contingent response reinforcement). However, in the third and fourth quarter of the first year, infants who have been ignored cry more often and they also cry longer, after mother has been there and has gone again, in those cases where mother's responses were habitually tardy. Mother's ignoring of the crying increases the likelihood of baby crying more often (and thus initiates a vicious cycle since mothers then ignore the crying infants more and more).

More important is that babies who cried little at the end of the first year had a wider range of communicative skills and more differentiated methods of eliciting responsiveness; mother's availability thus supported the development of social competence, even the early establishment of object permanence – the knowledge that objects exist even if they are not visible.

## (F) CONSTITUTIONAL MISMATCHING

There are many pitfalls in the delicately balanced mechanism of give and take between mothers and infants – a great deal may go wrong. The sensitivity of the mother to her baby is a crucial factor. There may be mismatching, which distorts the mutual relationship. Mothers may severely overload their child with signals – try to engage them in playful encounters when the child is not ready and turns away. They may then ignore the turning away and force the child's attention and the child finally resorts to tantrums and distress. If this continues the mother–child relationship may be permanently damaged. The fact that over-stimulation as well as under-stimulation may be damaging is often forgotten. Children in problem families are often over-stimulated: exposed to chaotic emotional experiences which they cannot understand.

There are also, according to Schaffer and Emerson (1964), children who actively resist physical contact, wriggle out of mother's arms if she tries to cuddle them. Mother, feeling rejected by the child, may then in turn reject the child herself. If this does not happen a bond may nevertheless be forged somewhat later, although initially it may be shallow: it becomes normal at 18 months, when the child's needs are satisfied by different methods (clinging to mother's skirt, following her with his gaze, etc.). On the other hand, absolute and perfect matching of mother–infant behaviour would be detrimental, since it is by adapting to new and unfamiliar situations and signals that the infant develops and learns; mothers therefore instinctively always slightly change their 'games' to retain the infant's attention.

Studies of babies with Down's syndrome have shown

some indication of abnormal child–infant interaction patterns in these early stages. These babies tend to repeat vocalizations more quickly, leaving little space for the dialogue. They also vocalize at the same time as mother more often than normal infants, clashing with her and showing lapses in interactive turn-taking skills. The most interesting fact which has emerged is, however, that children with Down's syndrome engage in the same rhythmic mutuality as normal children do, though mothers tend to be slightly more in control and show more initiative in the interaction with these children than with normal children. Nevertheless, even these children are clearly endowed with innate social skill and an innate need for communication, despite their slowness in learning.

## (G) INNATE SOCIAL DYSFUNCTION? AUTISM

Ricks' (1979) research with 7-month-old normal, autistic and retarded babies showed that normal as well as retarded infants gave specific sounds in specific situations which parents could recognize when the tape-recorded sounds were played back to them.

The vocal expressions in response to pleased surprise at a special event, the sounds uttered when a child is frustrated, when greeting a familiar person or when expressing a request are specific but similar in all normal and retarded infants, clearly conveying to the adult listener their specific message. These sounds seem to be part of the 'panhuman prespeech vocabulary'. However, autistic infants, though also responding with sound messages in specific situations, have sounds which are *not* recognized by adults and do not convey their meaning to outside listeners. They are consistent for each child, recognizable to those who live with them, but different from the sounds expected from normal infants and difficult to interpret.

Schaffer (1971), who based his findings about autistic

26

children on extensive interviews with the mothers, says that these children's ability to use 'signalling devices' is severely impaired during the early months of life. They may not cry at all when hungry so that mother has to guess whether she should feed and they may not make any sign of protest when adults leave the room. Moreover, Condon (1979), who scrutinized sound tapes of infants with different abnormalities, believes that in some infants the movements, which normally follow sound stimulation, occur either too late or too intensely, supporting the view that autistic babies are abnormal in processing the auditory modality.

None of these studies are entirely conclusive. However, autism – the puzzling condition of unknown aetiology which is hard to diagnose and which is often accompanied by mental defect, but may also occur in children of average intelligence – is more often found in middle-class than in working-class children (even when referring bias is taken into account). It is characterized, according to Rutter's (1976) criteria, by early onset of abnormality, impairment of social development, delayed language and insistence on sameness. It may be related to an abnormality in the inborn communicative mechanism which has come to light in the recent investigations.

The absence of social responsiveness in autistic babies has sometimes led to a false diagnosis of deafness, while on the contrary most of the autistic children are hypersensitive to noise – such as aeroplanes overhead and bangs. Nevertheless, they fail to listen when being talked to, or when called by their name. They do not acquire language at the appropriate time and abnormal language development is one of the essential symptoms of autism. Nevertheless, there are fundamental differences between children with a specific developmental receptive language disorder – the dysphasics – and the autistic children: the purely language-disabled child – just as the autistic – has difficulties in most aspects of language. Both groups are late, particularly in language comprehension, and in both groups one finds near relatives with language disorder. Both are often echolalic. However, the autistic's echolalia clearly indicates a lack of communicative intent, while the dysphasic child gropes for the meaning of what was said when echoing speech.

The autistic child's language deviation is most striking in those features which carry the emotional load of communication. His verbal disability – unlike the dysphasic's – extends over other aspects of communication: the understanding and imitating of gestures and social signs (Bartak *et al.* 1975) and it includes deviancy of 'inner language' and of imaginative and 'pretend play'. Moreover, gaze aversion is severe. There is rarely a fluctuating audiogram or poor sound discrimination, which is common in dysphasia.

Some autistics learn to talk and to communicate in a fashion; but their language remains almost invariably stilted, manneristic, monotonous in pitch and is characterized by the absence of the normal rhythm of speech. The children may take over entire chunks of adult speech, 'regurgitating' whole phrases: the child may call a kettle a 'make a cup of tea', and the confusion of pronouns so characteristic of autistic speech, which has previously been interpreted as denoting a confusion of identity, is part of this rigid takeover of entire chunks of adult speech. (It is described as a 'closed-loop phenomenon'.)

One of my autistic patients would say 'Jo must not have doctor's pen', when in fact what she wanted was to ask whether she could have my pen. At 3 years old she would confuse daddy and mummy linguistically. Many years later – having become a 'normal' schoolgirl, able to read and write and follow the school curriculum – she retained the original rigidity and lack of social empathy which characterized her previously. Aged 10 years, she would talk of her school as having 'a nice atmosphere', clearly having heard this phrase from adults, and she remained friendless, because according to her mother she would treat her age-mates as if *she* were their mother or teacher, adopting mannerisms inappropriate for her own situation. The only abnormality she is left with is an impaired social sense, a tendency to obsessive preoccupation with specific subjects for weeks or months.

Not many autistic children lose their strange communication pattern to the extent that this patient did (it is known that the condition is more common and more severe in males than females). Many develop organic symptoms such as epilepsy in adolescence and the likelihood of an organic basis to the illness has been supported by air encephalograms, where, in one research (Hauser *et al.* 1975) almost 90% of the children showed abnormalities in the temporal area. The likelihood of psychogenic origin (the so-called refrigerator mother), which had been asserted by some earlier workers (such as Kanner (1949) or Bettelheim (1967) ), is now largely refuted. It is not maternal deprivation which causes autism.

The clinician to whom the mother brings a 2-year-old, being puzzled about the child's strangeness and his lack of normal speech, will at this stage have no difficulty in diagnosing autism – failure to listen, gaze aversion, and bizarre response are indicators. A report from the mother of sudden, unexpected and inexplicable attacks of screaming panic which cannot be assuaged by distraction or cuddling will help confirm the diagnosis. Mother will sometimes say: 'But he can speak . . . he can count to 100. . . .' and will demonstrate this skill. But the child's speech is parrot-like; it is not symbolic. The prognosis is always tentative. The level of functioning in later life ranges from defective to almost normal. Many remain mute and in institutions, 20% have an IQ within the average range and, although most psychologists who test the children report back that the child's co-operation was too erratic to obtain a valid

IQ figure, the figure is the best predictor for the future. In one of the large series tested in the Maudsley Hospital, those with an IQ below 50 were not able to live in the community, while those with an IQ around 85 could function outside.

## (H) EARLY SOCIAL COMPETENCE AS A PREDICTOR FOR THE FUTURE?

If a child is seen earlier than one year, a careful observation of the play pattern between mother and infant, its rhythmicity and turn-taking synchrony, may give a valuable clue to the prognosis. We have recently learned a little about the predictive value of precocity in children who communicate with mother in particular harmony and this will be discussed in the next chapter.

It must be remembered, however, that developmental growth does not necessarily proceed in a straight line in the sense that the organism always builds on and elaborates what is known when younger. For instance, many of the skills of the newborn (such as walking, reaching, willingness to imitate adults, etc.) fade and must be relearned. One may therefore assume that similar situations may exist in social development with some social mechanisms fading and having to be relearned at a later stage – for instance, babies are born without fear of strangers, which develops after the first 6 months of life and has then to be unlearned. Mothers who can appreciate (Sameroff 1976) the discontinuous nature of the child's behaviour are better equipped to make changes in their handling as the child's activities and requirements change with development.

A mother's willingness to engage in a dialogue and to take her child's cues starts in the first days of life. This willingness to interact with her child, taking his cues as the instigator of her own response, should be strongly encouraged, whenever health visitors, nurses and midwives have a chance to do so, in view of its crucial effect on later development. Some mothers may wait for the permission by the expert before they dare to 'play' and 'have fun' with their child, rather than devoting their efforts to nappy-changing, feeding, cleaning and, later, teaching behaviours. Films showing mother–infant play might be highly interesting to expectant or young mothers when they visit antenatal or postnatal clinics. Talks about the importance for later development of intensive – not necessarily prolonged – turn-taking with babbles, smiles and gestures might be useful. J. and F. Newson (1979) say: 'Baby's best toy is her own mother: familiar yet changing, sometimes surprising – hard and soft ... a machine for bouncing, rocking ... with a most intricate sound mechanism.' Babies as well as mothers not only get joy from playing with each other; baby also learns in this way what animated objects can do and what can be done with them, an essential experience for later life.

# Chapter 2

---

# ATTACHMENT AND THE GROWTH OF FEAR

---

## (A) CONSTITUTIONAL FACTORS

The abnormality of pre-verbal communication with mother or care-taker, and the subsequent inability to establish social relationships with others, which is so characteristic of autistic children, strikes the observer as bizarre and puzzling. It is different from the asocial or antisocial behaviours of children with early conduct disorder which have also been postulated to be the consequence of disturbed early communication.

Separation of child from mother has often been said to be the cause of conduct disorder. While in autism the gross abnormality of social responsiveness is often evident before the sixth month and it is all-pervasive by 2 years of age, antisocial behaviour depends it is believed on events occurring *after* the sixth month when bonding begins in normals.

It is true that children who later develop disorders of the antisocial kind often show specific symptoms very early. There seems to be no doubt that there is an organic basis for 'sociability'. It was demonstrated by Freedman (1965) in his research on identical and fraternal twins. The babies were filmed from birth onwards month by month over the first year of life and the films were rated by independent observers who had never seen the children. Identical twins were far more concordant in their social responsiveness, in the amount of smiling and in the visual fixation of people than fraternal twins were. They were also more alike than fraternal twins in the amount of fear responses they exhibited after 6 months.

## (B) THE TEMPERAMENTAL ADVERSITY INDEX

Graham *et al.* (1975) studied children at risk in Camberwell, London, looking at those children where one parent had a psychiatric condition, and found that those children who, according to their mothers, had three specific features as babies tended to develop antisocial behaviours and conduct disorders one year later. These features were: first, intense and predominantly negative emotions (yelling rather than whimpering when in discomfort); second, they lacked rhythmicity of their bodily needs (mother could never predict when the child wanted to be fed, when it would want to sleep, etc.); and third, they were slow to adapt to new situations and were less fastidious and more tolerant of dirt than other children. The authors constructed a Temperamental Adversity Index and children high on this scale were eight times more likely than low scorers to develop behaviour disorders.

American studies (Thomas *et al.* 1968) in a follow-up of a group of 130 middle-class babies found that 20% of the children who would have been high on the Adversity Index were 'conduct disorders' in periods up to 5 years later. Studies still continuing reach similar preliminary conclusions.

It is, however, likely that environmental factors interact with these constitutional temperamental characteristics. Irregular irritable infants try a mother's patience and, if her capacity for giving is marginal, this trait may cause her to turn away from the child, who in turn feels 'unloved', thus laying the foundation for the alienation from their families typical for children and adults with antisocial behaviour. The paediatrician or the health visitor, nurse and family doctor may be able to explain the constitutional element to mothers and the consequences for the child of feeling unloved, thus preventing the establishment of a vicious cycle.

## (C) OBJECT PERMANENCE AND THE BEGINNING OF FEAR

In the normal child the vissicitudes of the 'attachment stage', assumed to begin at 6–8 months of life, are believed to be crucial for a child's social adjustment. Schaffer (1971) says: 'It is the development of the personal bond, of the ability to form differential relationships to specific individuals that constitutes the ultimate essential most intriguing aspect of early human behaviour. We tend to regard this as a *sine qua non* for mental health' and he goes on to ask, 'How does the infant form this primary relationship?' since the early communicative 'games' can be played by all and sundry, provided the partner is sensitive to the child's cues? What is the mechanism that brings about selective social behaviour?

During the first months of life the infant does not show any avoidance of unfamiliar people or objects. Smiles appear on his face in response to familiar sights after the second month and up to 3 months almost all infants smile indiscriminately at strangers. Some children may be able to discriminate between mother and others, perhaps even at 1 month of age, and though almost all children behave differently to mother and to strangers at 5 months of age, there is no avoidance of unfamiliar people. There is a delicate balance in the infant's make-up of preference for the familiar and counterbalancing need for novelty. The smile fades when situations or displays become repetitive and this is why mothers always slightly alter their singing, their words or their rhythms to retain the infant's attention. It is generally about the fifth month – sometimes earlier – that the infant begins to show wariness when unfamiliar persons approach him – he may frown or he may watch the stranger, as though he were comparing him with his mother – and his heart rate may decrease as a sign of attention and concentration. However, later his heart rate will increase when a stranger comes upon him and the child begins to show signs of fear – often quite suddenly.

At 8 months, according to the theories of Piaget (1955), object permanence is established: the child knows that a thing exists, even if it is not seen. In the first months of its life one may hide under a cup a little toy with which the baby has played. The baby may lift the cup where the toy is hidden: he will not grasp the toy, he will play with the cup – a thing, once it is out of sight, no longer exists for him. At 8 months, however, the baby will search with his eyes for a toy which has fallen out of the cot – and he will scan the surroundings in search. He remembers that toys do not vanish but exist even if they are not in view.

By this time the baby also knows that mother exists, even if she is not with him. He has, as it were, internalized mother's image; mother's absence is noted and the stranger is recognized as unfamiliar – he is unlike the mother's image which the child carries inside himself and he elicits fear in the baby when he tries to approach. Interestingly, monkeys reared in isolation (Sackett 1966) begin to show disturbed behaviours when, aged 60–80 days (not earlier), they are shown a picture of a monkey in threatening posture: 'the visual stimulation involved in threat behaviour functions as an "innate releasing stimulus" for fearful behaviour.' Spitz (1950) termed the infants' behaviour towards strangers in the second half of the first year of life the '8 months anxiety' though, in fact, the onset of fear reactions varies considerably from child to child and usually increases up to 2–2½ years.

The objects which elicit the greatest fears also change according to age (Table 1), and some fears wane after the

Table 1   Fears shown by children at various ages in experimental situations

| | Percentage of children showing fear | | | |
|---|---|---|---|---|
| *Situation* | *24–35 months* | *36–47 months* | *48–59 months* | *60–71 months* |
| 1.  Being left alone | 12.1 | 15.6 | 7.0 | 0 |
| 2.  Falling boards | 24.2 | 8.9 | 0 | 0 |
| 3.  Dark room | 46.9 | 51.1 | 35.7 | 0 |
| 4.  Strange person | 31.3 | 22.2 | 7.1 | 0 |
| 5.  High boards | 35.5 | 35.6 | 7.1 | 0 |
| 6.  Loud sound | 22.6 | 20.0 | 14.3 | 0 |
| 7.  Snake | 34.8 | 55.6 | 42.9 | 30.8 |
| 8.  Large dog | 61.9 | 42.9 | 42.9 | — |
| Total | 32.0 | 30.2 | 18.1 | 4.5 |

third year – there is a well-known pattern of fears of noise, loss of support, heights, strange people or objects, animals, the dark, etc. It is important to remember that at this time, from the eighth month onwards, hospitalization becomes an intense source of distress.

## (D) PATTERNS OF FEAR RESPONSES

Why does the unfamiliar elicit fear at this stage of a child's life? There is an interesting description of the fear of the unfamiliar in rhesus monkeys (Harlow and Suomi 1970). The rhesus monkey's 'cushion mother' – a contraption stuffed with cushions – usually had a painted doll's head made out of wood. At one time a rhesus baby arrived and the head was not ready. The experimenters placed a plain wooden ball on the surrogate mother's shoulders. To the baby monkey this featureless face became beautiful and the baby, from about 30–40 days of age, frequently caressed it with hands and legs. By the time the monkey had reached 90 days, the properly ornamented head was ready and mounted on the surrogate's body. The baby took one look and screamed, fled to the back of the cage and cringed in an autistic type of posturing. After some days of terror, the infant solved the problem of the medusa-mother by re-volving the face 180° so that it always faced the bare ball. When the face was turned again, the monkey resolved the situation finally: it lifted the maternal head from the body, rolled it into a corner and abandoned it. 'No one can blame the baby', say the experimenters, 'it had loved a faceless mother.' They concluded that the animal visually responds to the earliest version of the mother it encounters, and any changes after fear responses have begun elicit intense anxiety.

Children commonly become frightened when mother appears in a wig or with spectacles (though masks alone are considered acceptable toys). Harlow and Suomi (1970) say that comparison should be made between their rhesus baby and human children with babysitters. The shock to an infant over 8 months old on awakening and suddenly seeing the strange face of a babysitter may be traumatic. Harlow and Suomi, however, did not consider that a far more fundamental change of mother's image occurs in adoption and that this change may well cause intense upset. I shall return to the question of the change in mother's image in adoption later, when separation is discussed.

## (E) FIRST ATTACHMENT TO PEERS

Hunt (1964) says children try to retain situations they have repeatedly encountered. Fear responses develop slowly. The intensity of the fear increases as the distance from the strange object diminishes and is at its most intense when an adult stranger tries to touch the child. Unexpectedly, however, the child's fear is almost absent when the same procedure is adopted, not by an adult, but by another child. Size is not the decisive factor, according to experiments reported in Schaffer (1974). Adults of small size are feared as well, and it may be that children, even under 1 year of age, can discriminate between children and grown-ups and it seems that even at this young age there exists a rudimentary concept of identity of an idea of the self or 'like me'.

There is now a growing amount of literature suggesting that the importance for a child's development of relations with non-adults is far more essential than had been guessed. It was, of course, known for a long while that the non-human primates, such as the rhesus monkey, develop most bizarre and pathological behaviour if reared in isolation from peers (Figure 5). It had been assumed that this pathology was 'incurable', until experiments were started to bring younger, non-threatening monkeys to the withdrawn 'isolates'. The isolates would learn social skills by watching and playing with these younger monkeys and they began to acquire those skills which they had been unable to learn at the normal times. These experiments drew the attention of social psychologists to the interesting and important influence on the growing infant of peers and non-adult companions.

The most striking description of attachment to peers was that by Freud and Dann (1951). They reported the fate of six concentration-camp children who were separated from their parents from the age of 6 months and, after

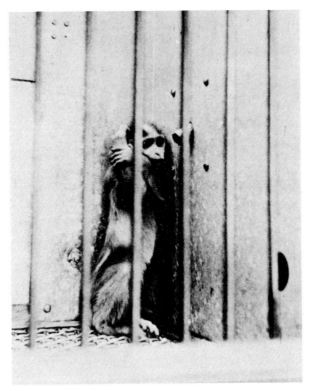

Figure 5   Behaviour of rhesus monkey 'isolate' [repro-
duced from *Friendship and Peer Relations* (ed. Lewis and
Rosenblum, 1975), p. 165, John Wiley & Sons, Inc., New
York, by permission of the publishers and the University
of Wisconsin Primate Lab.]

many vicissitudes in wartime Europe, reached England at
5 years of age. They were restless and uncontrollable but
their extensive contact with each other had produced a
high degree of mutual attachment. There was no evidence
of sibling rivalry. 'They had no other wish than to be
together and became upset when they were separated even
for short moments. No child would consent to remain
upstairs while the others were downstairs or vice versa,

and no child could be taken for a walk or an errand without the others. If anything of the kind happened, the single child would constantly ask for the other children, while the group would fret for the missing member.' This group of children clearly had come through a rare constellation of deprivation, but their behaviour shows that in extraordinary circumstances attachment to peers can to some extent replace the normal attachment to parents.

However, even where parents are normally available and attachment and bonding has occurred, the normal child is nevertheless in need of the companionship of non-adults for optimal social development. The urban Western society is quite 'unnatural' in its organization: parents with children below 18 months fail to encourage companionship with other children, except where there are siblings; whereas infants are socially inquisitive, preferring babies to adults, and community doctors or health visitors who see such isolated infants should recommend attendance at play groups at an early age. Children under 2–3 years of age do not play with other unfamiliar children, but they watch other infants with intense interest and positive affect, while their affect toward unfamiliar adults is negative (Figure 6) (Hartup 1980). Children aged 9 years speak 'motherese' with 2-year-olds, suggesting a natural empathy even of young children with younger infants.

Even when in play groups, toddlers do not truly interact; they have a common interest in toys and they learn to master manipulative tasks by watching each other. It is in the next stage that children begin to form affective encounters. Nevertheless, they are still inept at relating to each other. Konner (1975) asserts that integration of children into multi-age groups is essential for their development: 'peer relationships are artifacts of child-rearing conditions in industrial societies and the organization of schools and universities in western culture, strictly segregated by age, clearly has disadvantages for the learning of social skills

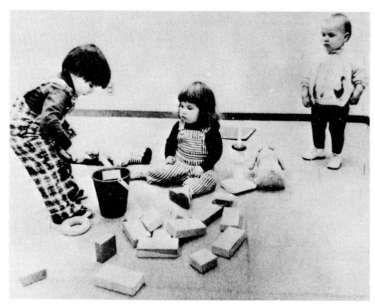

Figure 6    18-month-old child watching others at play
[reproduced with permission from *Friendship and Peer
Relations* (ed. Lewis and Rosenblum, 1975), p. 30, John
Wiley & Sons, Inc., New York]

which we tend to overlook.' It is, as Bronfenbrenner (1979)
points out, a severe handicap that in the urban culture
young women never have practice with bringing up small
babies or helping with infant rearing; they are therefore
badly prepared for parenting, overanxious when handling
their first baby, too self-conscious to engage in spontaneous
'motherese' – the vocal communication which is repetitive,
rhythmic, slow and accompanied by exaggerated facial
expressions. Having spent most of their lives – at kindergarten, in school, clubs and colleges – with same-age children, they have never helped to care for mother's younger
children and never helped to prepare food for the newborn
sibling or to bathe him; tasks which are natural in rural
and primitive communities (Figure 7). These girls tend to

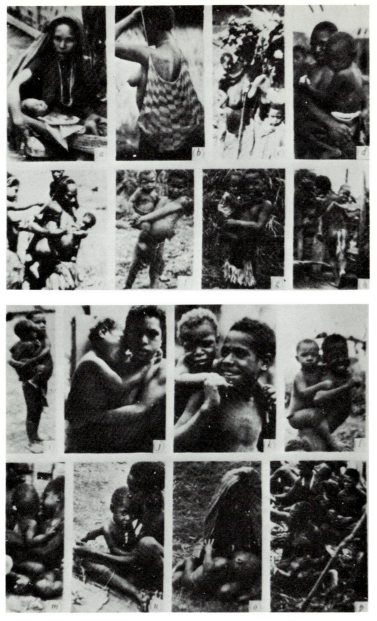

Figure 7   Early tactile communication in a New Guinea communmity [reproduced from *Before Speech* (ed. Bullowa, M., 1979), p. 296, Cambridge University Press, by kind permission of the publishers and Dr E. Richard Sorenson]

miss their own baby's signals once they have become mothers themselves. Bronfenbrenner adds: 'No society can long sustain itself, unless its members have learned the sensitivities, motivations and skills involved in assisting and caring for other human beings.'

# Chapter 3

## SEPARATION EXPERIENCES

### (A) THE ETHOLOGICAL ARGUMENT

Bowlby in his monograph *Maternal Love and Mental Health* (1951) and in his later publications, including *Attachment and Loss* (1969, 1973 and 1980), has influenced our thinking for the past decades about the way the child attaches itself to its mother.

Bowlby puts forward a theory of attachment and bonding where the early attachments are seen as the precursors of all social relations. Influenced by ethological theories of imprinting and following behaviour in animals, he believes that the infant is born with a biological propensity to behave in a way which promotes proximity and contact with his mother. As long as the infant is immobile, this is done by the social smile or by crying, which elicits mother's need to hurry to the child. Bowlby asserts that attachment behaviour in most mammals has as its goal the protection from predators. He implies innateness in the same way in which the monkey develops a fear reaction when seeing threatening pictures. Bowlby suggests that 'proximity-promoting' behaviour will be automatically activated when information reaches the infant that it has moved too far away for protection, and in the manner of a feedback loop attachment behaviours will be reinstated until proximity is re-established. Mother responds to the child's endeavour by cuddling, protecting, 'loving'. Bonding – which is permanent – develops as a consequence of maternal responsiveness to the child's needs.

## (B) MONOTROPY?

Many of Bowlby's assertions have proved correct though the ethological argument has been attacked and new investigations have modified some of his assertions. These are summarized by Rutter (1979a).

Bowlby believes that only mothers can provide the necessary response to the child's needs, and he formulated this in his famous (1951) dictum: 'Mother love in Infancy and Childhood is as vital to a child's mental health as protein and vitamin for his physical health.' Researches have demolished this theory of 'monotropy'. It is not *mother's* love alone which the child needs. The child may be attached to father (30% of English children, according to Schaffer (1964), have a closer tie to father than to mother), they may even be attached to non-human objects (like the rhesus monkeys to their 'mothers' constructed of cushions). Although there does exist in children a hierarchy of attachments (even children in institutions have a 'favourite' nurse), the attachment to all these figures, though varying in intensity, does not differ in kind. In primitive societies, as described by Margaret Mead (1962), there is always multiple mothering with no ill effect.

## (C) SEPARATION IN BROKEN FAMILIES

Bowlby believed that any separation from the figure of attachment was universally disastrous; particularly, that the so-called 'affectionless' character, the prototype of the psychopath, was shaped during prolonged separation from the person with whom the essential bond had been forged during the first year of life.

Investigations have shown that, indeed, conduct disorders in children often occur in broken homes but Rutter (1979a) asserts that this happens not because of the separation as such, but because of the disharmony and discord prior to the break-up of the home. It is not found to the same extent in children whose home broke up because of a death, although this, too, causes separation. Affectionless psychopathy, Rutter (1979a) says, is associated with an initial failure to form bonds and conduct disorder occurs more often in children who live in families with continued marital conflict than in those families where divorces have taken place. When counselling families, this point must be borne in mind; it must also be remembered that children with mothers who go out to work are not at risk as long as the substitute care is good and permanent. I shall discuss this important point later.

## (D) HOSPITALIZATION

The work of Bowlby (1946, 1951) and his collaborators asserted that separation of infant from mother was always unnatural, always disastrous and fundamentally always detrimental to healthy development. This assertion had, as its most far-reaching consequence, a new attitude towards children in hospital and in institutions. A large amount of literature has since accumulated and much research has been carried out. Bowlby's theories have been partly accepted and partly rejected.

Children who are whisked into hospital - often without being properly prepared for it, sometimes too young to understand any explanation - are immensely distressed. Bowlby (1979) and the Robertsons of the Tavistock Clinic (1967-72), who have filmed children in hospital during short-term and long-term separation from mother, asserted that three sequential stages characterize the child's reaction during such a traumatic event. The recognition of the symptoms characteristic of each phase remains an urgent requirement for hospital staff who deal with children, from medical students to nurses, to doctors and consultants.

In the first phase, labelled 'protest', the child cries, shakes the cot, throws himself about and does not respond to nurses in a desperate attempt to prevent mother from leaving or to force her to return. This phase may last from a few hours to weeks and it is only the return of mother which can comfort the infant. The next phase, 'despair', is characterized by a reduction in physical movement, by monotonous crying and withdrawal from social contact, resembling the state of deep mourning. The third phase, 'detachment', appears to the nursing staff as an amelioration of the child's condition; he has 'settled in', he now plays with other children and with the toys provided for him and makes friends with all and sundry (just as the affectionless character described by Bowlby in his early writings (1946)). But Bowlby says this stage represents a definite break in the mother–child relationship: the child may not respond to mother when she visits, and when the child eventually returns home, he may pretend not to recognize it; he may be rebellious or excessively clinging, expressing anger about the separation or fear that it may recur. This is believed to have a lasting effect and may even result in a flattening of affect for good.

It is important for the treating doctor that he makes it clear to the parents that this stage of 'detachment' must be carefully handled, anger accepted as normal and rejection of the family seen as transient. Sleep disturbances, such as crying at night, or excessive clinging behaviour in daytime so that mother will not even be allowed to go alone to the bathroom without tears, will generally disappear. The ill effects of the separation can be prevented by acceptance of this stage as normal – if mothers are warned beforehand and know what to expect.

Researches have confirmed that these phases may occur

in children as young as 18 months and as old as 14 years. However, in contrast to Bowlby's early assertions, there was no confirmation of any correlation with later post-separation symptoms of duration of hospital stay and, although the younger child (with a peak of 3 years) seemed the most upset, there was no age-related difference in later behavioural problem. (Except for Douglas' (1975) researches, which seemed to confirm long-term consequences of early repeated hospitalization in adolescents. However, since it is the most disturbed family which is most likely to have a child frequently in hospital, the research results are not convincing and are contaminated with social problems.)

The Robertsons (1971) in more recent investigations have developed devices which may alleviate children's distress: they have demonstrated how to prepare them for the experience, how to keep the bond with the home alive – by visits, photographs and familiar toys – and they have demonstrated that the separation does not necessarily leave long-term marks. Recent publications, funded by the National Association for the Welfare of Children in Hospital, have added advice about measures beyond those emphasized by the Robertsons: Landsdowne (1981) says that the experience of strangeness, the different beds, the people in uniform clothes, etc. are particularly upsetting to children and should be mitigated by familiarizing the child through play with what he is likely to meet when going to hospital. This should be done while the children are healthy, since, by the time they reach the age of 7, half of all children in this country will have spent some time in hospital.

Films are now available for showing to children before operations: they see the preceding procedures and watch another child of the same age deal with the experience. The NAWCH books show children having X-rays (Figure 8), having blood samples taken and being examined by doctors; they are illustrated, as realistically as possible, by

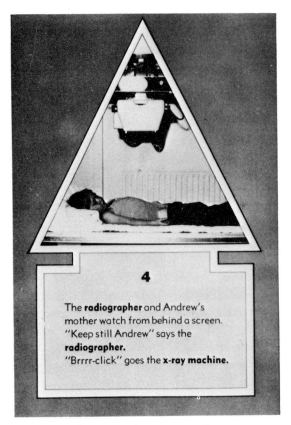

**4**

The **radiographer** and Andrew's mother watch from behind a screen. "Keep still Andrew" says the **radiographer**. "Brrrr-click" goes the **x-ray machine.**

Figure 8    A page from *Andrew Goes for an X-ray*, a book designed to reassure children visiting hospital [reproduced by kind permission of NAWCH]

photographs, with the idea that they should form part of children's books. Parents often share their children's anxieties about hospitals and doctors, and they, too, should be familiarized with the hospital by visits to the wards and by talking with the staff before the child's admission. Parents should be warned not to tell their children soothing lies such as 'a nice place where they make you better ... it won't hurt, etc.' Children will become distrustful with their parents when they later find that hospital is not only a strange place but that pain is often unavoidable. Moreover, nurses should learn to adjust hospital routine – including meal times, choice of food etc. – in such a way that life is more like that at home for the children.

Many of the Platt Report's recommendations are based on insights gained by the Bowlby team. Measures were instituted aimed at alleviating children's distress, such as unrestricted visiting, mother-in-units (where mothers stay in hospital wards with their children), etc. Researches have shown that these measures are indeed beneficial but their effect is not so convincing that they confirm Bowlby's theory that *any* separation of mother and child is uniformly disastrous. Rutter (1979a) says that the separation is a precipitant rather than an essential factor in the child's distress, in accordance with the revision of Bowlby's ethological thesis, which was recently formulated by the Swansea team in *Beyond Separation* (Hall and Stacey 1979), who assert that the separation hypothesis is 'too simple and too generalized'.

The impact of hospitalization on children is very varied: it is disastrously distressful for some children and can be weathered by others who are of equal age receiving the same treatment in the same length of stay in hospital. Hall and Stacey (1979) say: 'Although separation is an important factor in the antecedent of upset following hospitalization, it is not a sufficient factor.' The ill effect is due not to the disruption of the mother–infant bond but to the disruption of the child's social life, when he is uprooted from the family and friends: more and more the emphasis in child development research is placed on the importance of the social network in which the child lives.

The Swansea team has isolated factors characterizing the 'vulnerable' child, who is most likely to suffer most from hospitalization: research was carried out on 5–6-year-old children who spent 5–6 days in hospital for tonsillectomy: the vulnerable child was the one who was generally most involved with its own family, rarely played outside, had no interest in people except those in the family circle, had a close but ambivalent relationship with the siblings and generally had an anxious mother. The team also observed children in long-term stay – who suffered from orthopaedic conditions or asthma – and severely criticized the conventional hospital wards: such wards constitute an emotionally deprived environment. Their atmosphere creates feelings of uncertainty and mystery which upsets children. This atmosphere fails, above all, to provide the opportunity for the formation of permanent bonds; nor does it allow the maintenance of bonds formed before the child came into hospital.

## (E) PARENTING

There is, according to Ainsworth's researches (1974), a vital difference between secure and insecure attachment and this will be discussed in the next chapter, dealing with the way the infant gains independence from his mother. The question arises as to which parents facilitate the formation of the permanent bond. Its intensity is not dependent on the duration of interaction with the child and does not depend on the amount of stimulation provided – as mentioned before, over-stimulation may even be bad. The sensitivity to the individual child's needs is the essential factor. However, certain research data suggest that there may be other factors which influence bonding, although their exact relevance is uncertain.

Parents who have had poor experiences in their own childhood are least able to engage in sensitive interaction with the child. There are unavoidable occurrences in the neonatal period, such as separation of child and mother due to the need of the child to be kept in an incubator, which may distort an early relationship. Fifty-nine young mothers, expecting their first child and interviewed before delivery, reported that they had been separated from either of their parents before the age of 11 years; 6 months after delivery they were shown to be less able to manage their babies than a control group of non-separated mothers, matched in all other respects. They breast fed for a shorter period, many stopped attending clinics, the babies had more sleeping problems, etc. (Frommer and O'Shea 1973).

There is a famous study by Klaus and Kennel (1976), showing that mothers who had immediate contact with their infant after delivery have different ways of handling their babies one month afterwards than those mothers where hospital routine was followed. The differences were still evident 1 year later. The experimental group had the baby for 1 hour immediately after delivery and 5 extra hours on each of the next 3 days. The other mothers had a brief contact with their babies 6–8 hours after delivery and then 20–30 minutes for feeding every 4 hours. The mothers in the experimental group were more affectionate to their babies and kissed and cuddled them more than the other mothers did. A study made in the Radcliffe Infirmary in Oxford, aimed at confirming these observations, found the same distinct difference in interaction with the infant between the two groups. The mothers who had no opportunity to handle the newborn for any length of time in hospital were less able to play with the infant when they came home. However, in this instance the difference disappeared after 4 months.

Another effect of early contact between mother and her newborn still more striking because it lasted only 20 minutes is reported by De Chateau (1980): a group of mothers were given their newborn for 20 minutes directly after delivery and the naked baby was placed in the suckling position during this period. It is claimed that even after 1 year, mothers who had this experience demonstrated greater enjoyment of their infants (mainly of their boy children) than the controls did. There was more cuddling and breast feeding was prolonged. However, interestingly some mothers outrightly refused the offer of such early contact and the author suggests that there may be a sensitive early post-delivery phase of which midwives and obstetricians should be aware.

Interesting in this context is the result of a questionnaire recently put to mothers about their feelings for their baby just after delivery. Robson and Moss (1970) report that they interviewed 54 primiparae mothers who said that strong feelings of attachment were not present in them until the baby's third month. 34% said the first contact elicited no feelings and Packer and Rosenblatt (1979), from observation of newly delivered children, say that 18% of mothers never looked at their infant after delivery, though they discussed him with their husbands, and only *half* of the mothers talked to their infants. The paediatrician may keep these studies in mind when it becomes necessary to allay guilt feelings of mothers who come to blame themselves for problems which arise with the baby later on.

The team working on the Harvard Preschool Project under the guidance of Burton (1979) has just published its final findings on the result of training and investigating parenthood behaviours. After a lengthy pilot project they followed up their children – 15 in the experimental group and 45 in control groups – with constant home visiting, interviewing and testing from 7 months to 18 months. A final assessment was made at 3 and $4\frac{1}{2}$ years, taking care that the families were within the 'average' range in every respect. The most surprising finding was the extent to which parents' treatment of their first-born differed from that of any subsequent children. These first-born received more attention, were provided with more appropriate surroundings and their final assessment showed their superiority over those born later.

The team believed that they had found three areas in

which successful childrearers excelled. Firstly, the children were given appropriate space in which to move freely with interesting toys appropriate to their size which they could explore at levels they could reach. Secondly, mother was available to them whenever they needed comfort or explanation, and they shared their excitement. Thirdly, successful childrearers disciplined and controlled their children firmly and consistently. On the strength of their experiences the team has set up a Centre for Parent Education where professionals are trained to work with young adults, to teach them child-rearing patterns. The researchers maintain that in this important area expert guidance should be available to parents; one may, however, doubt the effectiveness of such methods! Learning is best done by serving an apprenticeship – not by words. Experience should be given to all future parents in the handling and enjoyment of babies and infants, and girls and boys in the upper classes of secondary schools might – as part of their curriculum – be provided with opportunities to play with children in the infants' classes or to work in children's hospitals, in kitchen or wards where they can watch the nursing of babies and the contact of parents with their newborn.

## (F) ADOPTION

The relevance for adoption policy of most of the researches on separation is clear. Yarrow and Goodwin (1974) report on 70 adoptions (Table 2). At no age are infants completely insensitive to the changes in the environment associated with a change from a foster home to an adoptive home. The least severe disturbance occurred in those adopted below 3 months of age, where the upset clearly was caused by the change in the environment and routine but not by the loss of the foster-mother. In nine children under 3 months only five showed some disturbance, three of them

# Social development

Table 2   Reactions to adoption

| Age of placement (months) | Major areas of disturbance (% of all cases) | | | | | Total no. of cases |
|---|---|---|---|---|---|---|
| | Feeding | Sleep | Social | Emotional | Drop in IQ | |
| 1–3 | 0 | 11 | 0 | 11 | 23 | 9 |
| 3–4 | 10 | 30 | 30 | 20 | 60 | 10 |
| 4–5 | 22 | 44 | 28 | 17 | 39 | 18 |
| 5–6 | 27 | 53 | 47 | 27 | 47 | 15 |
| 6–7 | 43 | 71 | 57 | 43 | 50 | 7 |
| 7–9 | 60 | 80 | 80 | 80 | 50 | 5 |
| 9–12 | 67 | 67 | 100 | 68 | 0 | 3 |
| 12–16 | 25 | 50 | 25 | 50 | 0 | 3 |

From *The Competent Infant* (eds. Stone, Smith and Murphy, 1970, p. 1033), by kind permission of Tavistock Publications Ltd, London

mild. By 4 months, however, there was a clear change: 72% showed moderate to severe reactions. Some of them – below the 6-month stage – became withdrawn and apathetic, reminiscent of the description by Spitz (1946) of the dramatic illness (he termed it anaclitic depression) which happened in 6-month-old institutionalized children. They stopped eating, became utterly unresponsive, lost weight and had frozen, expressionless faces until mother returned. In children adopted after 6 months there was either a general change in social responsiveness, apathy, exaggerated stranger anxiety, feeding problems, sleeping disturbance, colics, etc., or even directly negative reactions to the new mother compared with the foster-mother. The child became tense and rigid when handled by the adopting mother and refused to be soothed. Some became excessively clinging. Three children who had been adopted after 9 months had the most severe problems with adjustment.

Counselling future adopters, which is often the clinician's duty, must take account of these findings: of the probably innate propensity of the human to react with fear and disturbance to changes in the care-taker. The counsellor must be aware of the varied forms these disturbances may take: somatic or behavioural symptoms may appear and it is important to be sensitive to the possible reaction of the new care-taker to a difficult child. The timing of the adoption is an important factor and, if possible, a bond should be preserved if it has been formed before adoption. With all these warnings, however, the developmental paediatrician must remember that the idea of the irreversibility of the effects of early adverse experiences has been challenged (Clarke and Clarke 1976). The effects of early experiences are no longer believed to be irreversible, unless subsequent events reinforce the early adversities, and Tizard's researches (1976) show that children, adopted after 4 years, have developed close relationships with the adopted parents as late as 4–6 years (though the children continued to show some social and attention problems at school).

Tizard's experiences have led her to believe that it is wrong to postpone adoption for too long in the hope that the natural mother will eventually reclaim the child to take it to live with her until adulthood. The adopted children had significantly fewer problems than those who stayed in the institution after 4 years even where the institutions have an excellent staff–child ratio, because it is difficult to ensure continuity of care with inevitable staff changes.

The idea that it is the natural mother who in every case is the best person to care for her child has been shown to be a myth rather than a reality. Doctors being consulted about care orders can exert a most beneficial influence in court, pointing to the evidence that, where a parent is unsatisfactory, alternative placement (perhaps eventually leading to adoption or permanent fostering) is preferable.

Quinton (unpublished observations 1981) has reported on a continuing study at the Maudsley Hospital of girls who had been in care and are now grown up: two-thirds of the 44 girls, taken into care aged $3-3\frac{1}{2}$ years, have now, as adults, no current psychiatric problem; one third of them did badly. Teachers' ratings were valid predictors for outcome in all areas except later parenting. Subsequent events occurring after the care order had the most decisive influence: those girls who went back to a good family were in the 'good outcome' group, while parenting problems were present in the 'bad outcome' group and correlated little with adverse experiences in the early years.

# Chapter 4

# FIRST STEPS TO INDEPENDENCE

## (A) THE RELEVANCE OF THE SOCIAL HISTORY

Before investigating a child's condition on being seen for the first time in the clinic, the developmental paediatrician naturally inquires carefully as to prior events, possibly relevant to the present state, particularly if it concerns failure to thrive, unexplained injuries, scars, etc. An important part of this fact-finding procedure is the social history: a detailed look at the child's social environment and development. Who was the main person involved as care-taker when he was tiny? Did the child respond to the mother's play and smiles? The questions will not only aim at excluding sensory, auditory or visual defects, but also attempt to assess possible social deviance of the child; answers may perhaps point to sudden changes in responsiveness – such as occur after separation. This may be relevant to the present complaint or may point to long-standing problems. How often and how sudden were separations from the figure of attachment? How long was the separation, and was there a sibling born when the condition developed? (Separations are the rule and not the exceptions in our culture.) Who looked after the child in mother's absence? Has the child pre-sleep rituals – suggesting a need to banish fears of being left alone at night?

Has he nightmares after, perhaps, toilet training? Above all, has the child established a secure bond to any one person or is this bond insecure?

## (B) THE VICISSITUDES OF ATTACHMENT BEHAVIOUR

Ainsworth *et al.* (1971) have described in detail the fundamental difference between attachment behaviour – proximity seeking, which is increased by anxiety, illness and even by rejection – and bonding, which allows the child to abandon the mother or care-taker's proximity, to explore novel objects and situations in the certainty that she will be there in case of danger. The child knows that mother will be available and responsive when he returns. The security of bonding and the ensuing readiness of the child to venture into the world – with occasional glances towards the mother – is the second important step in social development. It is one of the principal functions of mother to free the child once it is mobile and able to communicate by speech with her over distance. On the strength of the internalized image of the mother depends the child's ability to grow up. According to Ainsworth's hypothesis, the mother's sensitivity to the child's needs is the decisive factor in the child's readiness to leave.

Bowlby, elaborating his theory of attachment and bonding, emphasized that bonding is permanent, while attachment behaviour is activated only occasionally, particularly during stressful events, even in adolescents. The basic pattern is, he believes, under genetic control; vicissitudes are due to the environment. Ainsworth's (1974) experiments describe three types of attachment on the strength of her experience: the *securely* attached child who is active in play, even with strangers, and seeks contact with the mother only when in distress; the *anxiously* attached child who is in fear of strange situations and feels insecure even when mother is accessible; and finally the *attachment re-sistant* child who sometimes seeks contact and sometimes not. Bowlby in a recent unpublished paper (1980) says that researchers show a clear continuity between these three forms of attachment and the personality dimensions of ego-control and ego-resilience measurable in later life.

The *securely* attached child has 'moderate' ego control – i.e. he is not impulse-ridden, does not lack control, nor is he over-controlled – his ego resilience is high, he is resourceful and has a sense of competence. The *anxiously* attached child is too high in ego control and lacks spontaneity, while the *non-attached* child is far too little controlled and his ego is brittle – he tends to develop conduct disorders. Attachment behaviour is intensified by anxiety and by stress; strangely enough, even maltreatment by the figure of attachment increases the proximity-seeking behaviour of the child. Feeding and duration of contact with the figure of attachment are irrelevant and active reciprocal interaction between child and mother, if they are together, is of immense importance. Many investigators, among them Rubinstein (1967), found that the more often mothers looked at and talked to their babies, the more often and intensely their babies explored and manipulated objects and situations. Babies whose mothers were rated 'high-attention' mothers vocalized three times as much as those with 'low-attention' mothers. Yarrow *et al.* (1971) found in an investigation of 10-year-old adopted children that the depth of relating to others, social dominance and social effectiveness at 10 years were significantly related to early maternal communication, positive emotional expression, and appropriateness of stimulation received at 6 months.

There is, according to Ainsworth *et al.* (1974), a 'dynamic balance between exploratory and attachment behaviour, significant from an evolutionary point of view'. Attachment behaviour serves a protective function, while exploratory behaviour reflects the biological need of an

infant to be interested in the novel features of his environment, to approach them, to learn about the nature and
property of objects. This is not unique to the human species
and is also observed in non-human primates.

## (C) THE EXPLORATION OF THE WORLD

Exploratory behaviour, the learning of, on the one hand,
what things in the environment can do, and, on the other
hand, how many things one can do with them, is the basis
for creativity, for the ability to make novel responses.
Piaget says 'the more a child has seen and heard, the more
he wants to see and hear'. But there are children in whom
the smooth balance between attachment and exploratory
behaviour is upset and in Stayton *et al.*'s (1971) studies
such deviance was clearly associated with mother's attitudes, rated along the dimensions of sensitivity–insensi-
tivity, acceptance–rejection, accessibility–ignoring and
co-operativeness–interfering.

The children of the rejecting, the interfering, or ignoring
mothers displayed abnormal patterns in this balance, so
essential for social functioning. Where the child is secure
in his knowledge that mother will be available to him in
distress, separation will not have a permanent effect. It will
not engender distrust anxieties, etc. Separation *may* leave
permanent emotional scars, when the child is insecure
about mother's availability. Even in rhesus monkeys
similar differences can be shown to exist. I will return to
this when I discuss problems related to the child's integration into the wider world of peer groups in school and
schoolphobia, where the security or insecurity of the child's
bond to his home is a vital factor.

## (D) THE GROWTH OF OBEDIENCE

It is at the end of the first year that mothers begin to issue verbal commands: 'Don't do this …', 'go …', 'leave it alone', etc. (Though the child does not understand the words, he clearly understands their meaning by tone of voice and context.) Obedience to such commands and internalization of prohibitions (not to touch the radiator, not to splash water, etc.) is essential for the child's protection and it is at the core of his social behaviour later on. Richards (1974) believes that a disposition to be obedient is an essential manifestation of the normal infant–mother relationship, but that anomalies occur as the quality of mother's care deviates from the ideal. He studied 26 children and found that in the first year of life 86% of the children of 'sensitive' mothers obeyed commands, while only 49% of the infants of less sensitive mothers did. The clinician will probably have to include in his social history questions such as: 'Does he obey commands? Yours? His father's?', etc.

The observation of the child's natural tendency to obedience fits into the ethological argument. Infants (even in the animal world) engaged in the exploration of their surroundings must obey signals emitted by the figure of attachment as a safeguard against danger. Obedience and locomotor exploration appear in human children at the same time. As the infants move about to investigate, mothers must be able to control their actions across an often hazardous environment. Development of compliance with mother's signals therefore confers a biological advantage.

If, indeed, obedience is a natural inborn tendency, it follows that the kind of discipline exerted by the care-taker has little influence on the child's behaviour. This has been documented by experimental observations (Stayton *et al.* 1971): harsh or soft demands, reward for good behaviour and punishment for non-compliance influenced the small child very little at the early stage of development. Even the threat of 'loss of love', postulated as so important in inducing the child to behave well, seemed irrelevant. It is in those mother–child couples which are most harmonious and where 'loss of love' is least likely that obedience developed best: mothers who were most sensitive to the infant's signals, most accepting of his needs, and least restrictive and interfering had infants who followed their commands most unquestionably, at the ages between 9 and 12 months. Physical control by their mothers was least needed by these infants. On the other hand, rejecting mothers or those who interfered most with the child's activities, disregarding their needs, had children who were least compliant.

This experimental observation suggests not only that disciplinary practices are not related to obedience, but also that a disposition towards compliance emerges in responsive social environments without extensive training and without massive attempts to shape the infant's behaviour. It has an important bearing on the fundamental theoretical problem of social developmental psychology, which is concerned with the processes disposing children to act in accordance with the values and prescriptions of society. If special intervention is, indeed, not needed, to modify an assumed asocial child, the development of an initial disposition towards compliance may be a critical factor in the effectiveness of all further socialization. A child who lacks this fundamental tendency might be expected to remain in many ways a stranger to his culture.

However, in the second year of life there emerges commonly a tendency to negativism, which must be understood as the child's first attempt to develop independence – a 'will of his own'. It may very well depend on the successful handling of this first tendency to disobedience whether the next step of 'socialization' – toilet training – can be achieved without friction.

## (E) FIRST SOCIAL DEMANDS: TOILET TRAINING; ENURESIS AND ENCOPRESIS

In demanding that the child control its eliminatory functions, use the pot or the lavatory, when asked to do so, the parent for the first time requests something which has no protective aim, but is dictated by social convention and needs. Correct timing of this step is essential.

Bladder control may begin any time between 18 and 20 months – early potting has no influence on its success – but delay beyond the twentieth month, according to Shaffer *et al.* (1980) increases the likelihood of enuresis. Enuresis is 'normal' up to 3 years, but delay beyond this time is usual in retarded children while, according to the National Child Development Study (Davie *et al.* 1972) persistent enuresis during the day should be regarded as abnormal after the age of 3 and bed-wetting after the age of 4. In this study (comprising 1600 children, born during one week in March 1958 in Britain) mothers reported that one in nine of the children wetted their beds after the age of 4.

Enuresis is common in children with delayed speech and more common in boys than girls (12% against 10% in the NCD study). Girls mature faster. Nocturnal enuresis increases to 12–15% at 7 years, when entrance to junior school causes anxieties. In favour of a biological aetiology of enuresis, experts quote the facts that 15% of enuretic children have relatives with the same complaint and monozygotic twins are more concordant in this respect than fraternal twins are. Moreover, many enuretic children have a so-called 'irritable' bladder, i.e. they vacate the bladder in daytime before it is fully extended. However, it is difficult to say how far these symptoms are due to social and psychological causes (an irritable bladder may be caused by anxiety and tension) and it is certain that there are psychosocial factors in most cases. It is more common in disadvantaged groups, in large families, in institutions and in children with adverse experiences during their first years. Experience of stress during the time when continence is usually acquired may lead to persistent incontinence. For instance, $2\frac{1}{2}$–$3\frac{1}{2}$-year-old children reacted with regression in toilet training to the divorce of their parents with father leaving the family (Wallerstein and Kelly 1975). Clearly pointing to psychological causes is the fact that 20% of enuretic children are 'cured' by placebo treatment such as the visit to the doctor, the keeping of records and rewards for 'success'. (Frequent nightly lifting is not recommended since it teaches the child to vacate the bladder before it is full.) The higher incidence of enuresis at 7 years (as compared with 5 years) also shows its association with tension and anxiety (since it coincides with entrance to formal school).

Not all children who have failed to master bladder control by 3 years are emotionally disturbed, but most are. However, treatment for the emotional disorder is not always successful in stopping enuresis. Among the psychological reasons which may contribute is 'passive aggression' – a demonstration of anger against mother, who has to change sheets and clothes. Another reason may be the need for continued dependence (particularly when the next baby arrives and mother is observed changing the baby's nappies). It has also been said that wetting serves sexual gratification, but there is no difference in masturbatory behaviour between children with and without bladder control.

Treatment (if the child is free from any organic dysfunction or infection) consists of placebo cures, medication (unfortunately enuresis almost invariably reappears when the drug is stopped), and behaviourist methods such as the Bell and Pad, which is said to cure 90% of cases (but has a relapse rate of 35%). There is also systematic training in daytime; to increase the intervals between bladder emptying. There are also rather drastic training methods, mainly for very retarded children or adults. Persistent enuresis, particularly in girls above 10 years of age, is a danger signal and often precedes severe disturbance in adulthood.

Psychoanalytical theory always considered the period in which the child first tries to be independent as an important milestone in his development. In the 'anal' stage, the child sees the evacuated faeces as a 'gift'. The way the parents handle this phase, has, according to analysis, a vital influence on the child's future development. Their handling of this phase may lay the foundation for later severe abnormalities. It is sphincter control which for many parents seems to be the most important manifestation of a child fitting into society: a child who still soils, when his contemporaries are out of nappies, may upset mother no end. (Sphincter control normally starts at about 3 years of age and 1.2% of children still soil at the age of 7 years. Soiling is three times more common in boys than in girls.)

Children who soil longer than normal may come from chaotic families where training was neglected and soiling is 'continuous' until treated. In 'discontinuous' encopresis – i.e. in children who have been trained, but who occasionally fall back into soiling – the symptom is highly correlated with abnormally severe training by parents. Parents who over-emphasize cleanliness, who are obsessively preoccupied with toilet habits – often caused by their own childhood experiences (or even by guilt feelings about 'dirty' business in the literal and symbolic sense) – may become too severe when teaching the child how to use the lavatory: 63% of children with this kind of encopresis have been exposed to severe toilet training. Life in these families may centre on problems of cleanliness, and the child's anxiety about the problem may cause 'retentive' encopresis; the child becomes constipated, soils by 'overflow', initiating a vicious cycle of soiling, increasing the parents' anger thus increasing the child's fear to 'let go'. It may be the beginning of a battle between child and parent which may have serious consequences. Soiling as diarrhoea may also – just like in adults – be caused by anxiety, or may express anger.

It is significant that children often begin to soil again after toilet habits had been successfully established when a sibling arrives on the scene. Soiling may then be the only way for him to demonstrate to the parents his hidden aggressive feelings against the newcomer who is allowed to be a baby and act accordingly. I once showed an encopretic boy a test picture (Symonds' Tell a Picture Story Test) of a young woman flanked on each side by a little girl, and I requested him to tell a story. He said: 'This one has a birthday (the girl carried a flower). This one (the other girl) is angry, but she does not go to the toilet, she goes to the village, buys a gun and shoots this one (the adult).' An entirely unexpected confirmation of Freudian ideas – that toilet habits, anger and aggressive feelings are closely linked in unconscious fantasies.

Questions about toilet-training methods are clearly an important part of the social history and counselling about the best way of dealing with toilet training is one of the items which paediatricians discuss with parents of children at the toddler stage. The theory that children who soil will necessarily become compulsive, rigid adults has not been confirmed by scientific studies. Psychotherapy for both mother and child is nevertheless often the only method to prevent the relationship between parent and child becoming severely distorted and behaviour therapy for the soiling child, often successful, must be accompanied by help for the parent.

## (F) EARLY NEGATIVISM

How does one teach a child to cope with anger and aggressive feelings in a sociable, acceptable way? I have already mentioned important constitutional factors which may predispose a child to develop a so-called 'conduct disorder', manifest after the second and third year of life by defiance of rules, fighting, destructiveness, screaming, etc. There is evidence that children who show such negativistic features in the extreme do not usually 'outgrow' this phase, but tend to become difficult in school. On the other hand, there is a period during the second year when most children refuse to do whatever they are being told. They want to do things their own way and their most frequent word is 'NO'. They may refuse to be dressed, to have their hair washed, to be bathed, etc. Negativism and temper tantrums, when frustrated, are normal at this stage. They are at their peak at 2 years of age; not surprising at a time when a child, whose demands have always been gratified as long as he was helpless, becomes angry because suddenly his parents begin to consider him 'grown-up' and make demands accordingly. Often parents are at this period preoccupied with another baby.

By 3 years the tantrums become shorter and are followed by sulking, whining or brooding. By 4 years of age extreme negativism is generally overcome; however, personality difficulties of children or parents and features of the environment may reinforce and strengthen the negativistic phase, causing a vicious cycle of unruliness, punishment and anger, setting the stage for severe maladjustment and 'alienation' of the child from the family.

Failure or distortion of the socialization process may occur at different times, in different contexts and be caused by different factors. The label 'conduct disorder' may manifest itself in various ways – it is not a clear diagnostic category. It may represent an attempt by the child to control the parent – express aggressive rebellion against authority. It is called 'Tension-Discharge-Disorder' in one American nomenclature. It occurs three times as often in boys as in girls and only a small proportion of children with such disorder, leading to delinquent behaviour such as stealing, are ever seen by the courts. (70% of a random sample of 1425 London boys between 13 and 17 years old from all social-class levels admitted that they had stolen from shops.) An American study of 33 children aged 4 years who had no home problems and psychiatric disorders, demonstrated that the probablility was only 1 in 4 that the child would obey a command the parent gave him. Isolated antisocial or delinquent acts are so common that they are of little diagnostic significance; but if a child's conduct has unfavourable consequences, affects his learning ability, is constantly painful to others and deviates widely from social norms, parents rightly become concerned and these children are seen by clinicians.

Tolerance of conduct disorder varies widely in different families and negativistic behaviour may in some parents arouse such anger, resentment, feeling of helplessness and indignation that they react with counter-aggression, aggravating the situation.

Parents who bring their child, aged 3 or older, to the clinician because of the abnormal frequency of their child's antisocial acts or of the unbearable intensity of their yelling, screaming and stamping or of the sadistic flavour of their destructive and aggressive actions usually come with a negative mental set. They are eager to talk about their children's misdeeds and are almost unable to see anything good in them. They are in need of help for themselves as well as for the offspring. One of the first tasks of the counselling agent is to assist the parent in finding in the child positive features, some praiseworthy assets or efforts, which might be rewarded, so that the child's misdeeds can be 'punished' not by aggressive and negative means but by more positive action such as withdrawal of praise or reward. The clinician must remember the five factors conducive to the acquisition of rules by children noted by Wright (1971).

(1) Strong ties of affection between parent and child.
(2) Firm, clear demands made by the parents.
(3) The *consistent* use of sanctions.
(4) Punishments which are psychological rather than physical (physical punishment is least effective).
(5) Intense use of reasoning and explanation as soon as the child is ready for them.

## (G) SCHOOL REFUSAL

Normal children generally enter a 'conformist' stage, just before school age. However, some still find beginning formal education a major obstacle. In some of these children negativism may take the form of school refusal. All children, between $2\frac{1}{2}$ and 3 years, go through a phase of some misery when they first enter a nursery or play group and are left with strangers. They display signs of uneasiness and apprehension, tears are usual and tics may appear. They may stand and dreamily watch the others or reject the approach of older children. Some may refuse to speak for a long time in the presence of strangers and the (rare) condition of 'elective mutism' may become evident at this stage. It is difficult to treat and although it may disappear spontaneously, it can also continue until and beyond adolescence. After 4 weeks most children have adjusted. Some re-start the period of misery on entering the infant classes of junior school, but most, although they dislike school almost all of their lives, submit to the social demands to attend – and some may even in the end enjoy it.

After all, school is the first testing ground outside the protection of the home, requiring the need to submit to rules from which there is no escape. There is a chance of failure. One is exposed to judgements by others and one may be judged for features over which oneself has no control: one's looks, one's colour, etc. A few children are unable to accept the challenge and refuse to attend. School refusal is a severe condition – the child desires to conform to the social demands, but cannot do so. It occurs mainly at three different periods (Hersov 1977): between 5–7 years, at 11 years – the time of change to the secondary school – and at 14, in adolescence.

For a period physicians distinguished between school-phobia and truancy, assigning schoolphobia to the neurotic disorders and truancy to the behaviour disorders. The difference is now considered less clear cut. The schoolphobic child stays at home, unable to leave, may produce somatic symptoms, vomit and suffer from stomach cramps, headaches and tachycardia such that the parents don't dare to send him away, fearing that he may be seriously ill. (Children with stomach cramp, headaches, etc. may be recognized as schoolphobic by the fact that their symptoms don't occur on Saturday or during holidays.) The truant child, on the other hand, is said to leave for school, but may never get there or run out as soon as school starts. He roams the streets, until it is time to go home. Truancy as well as schoolphobia are now seen by some authorities as different forms of a complex collection of syndromes with different aetiology, prognosis, treatment and different degree of severity. The schoolphobic child generally comes from a neurotic family. He is often depressed, although frequently a good scholar.

The truant child is more afraid to face any challenging situations – he is scholastically backward and often somewhat delinquent. The prevalence is 17 in 1000 children with a peak period at 11 years, after the entrance to secondary school, but truancy may include as many as 10% of the 16-year-olds in some schools. (School refusal in adolescence is different from the condition in earlier years and we shall discuss this in a later chapter.)

In the younger child schoolphobia has been ascribed to 'separation anxiety'. It is certainly closely linked to the degree of security of bonding. Bowlby believes that the schoolphobic child is too frightened to leave a home where he cannot be certain that his mother will be there when he returns – he (1973) asserts that mother's threats to leave the child are more common than is ever admitted. Mother's separation anxiety is, according to Bowlby, also a potent factor in the syndrome since a child's schoolphobia often coincides with the death of mother's mother.

Hersov (1960), who interviewed 50 schoolphobic and 50 truant patients of the Maudsley Hospital, found that 18 of the young phobics admitted that their main fear was that some harm might befall the parents while they were out. There was, contrary to expectation, no increased incidence of early separation experience in the schoolphobic children, but half of the mothers had come from broken homes and an anxiety state of either parent often resulted in the child being kept at home. Neurotic illness in the parent is almost invariably present and needs treatment.

The great proportion of young schoolphobic children eventually return to school (89% of those under 11 years of age) but they need prolonged help, exploring the reasons and the kind of the child's fears. Perhaps a death among relations or friends, fear of a severe discord among the parents, or fear of teachers at school may have been the precipitant. Reality fears may be present in a tangle with unrealistic fantasies. Psychologists often use behaviour modification techniques or desensitization procedures, habituating the child by small steps to the situation which originally aroused his anxiety such as the assembly in school, playground, a specific teacher, etc. Treatment for the parents is almost always essential. Nevertheless, 50% of schoolphobics manifest neurotic symptoms in adulthood (and often have schoolphobic children). The clinician to whom the problem is presented must keep in mind the probable pathology of the parents and the circumstances in which the anxiety arose. And although depression is often present, treatment with anti-anxiety or antidepressant medication has not been effective (Berney *et al.* 1981). Eisenberg (1958) emphasizes the ambivalence of mothers who keep the child out of school: on the one hand, the child is a companion and relieves her loneliness; on the other hand, he imprisons her, watches her, impedes her freedom. The children themselves often timid and inhibited in school, show 'acting out' behaviour in the security of the home, being wilful, dominating and stubborn and the situation may have to be solved as quickly as possible to prevent further complication in the child-parent relationship.

## (H) CHILDHOOD REACTION TO PARENTAL LOSS BY DEATH OR DIVORCE

Bowlby's last volume of his trilogy *Attachment and Loss* (1980) describes the behaviour of children after the death of one parent and quotes many cases where schoolphobia is among the sequelae. It occurred, he says, in those frequent cases where the surviving parent 'inverts' the child-parent relationship, leaning on the child for comfort in bereavement. The child then becomes anxious about leaving the house; he may have overheard threats by the bereaved survivor that life is no longer worth living.

Bowlby is particularly explicit about the advice to be given to the surviving parent (or relative) who has to deal with a bereaved child of any age. He believes that contrary to previously held ideas, even very young children know from the observation of dead animals that death is final, that it is natural both to feel sad about it and to wish the dead would be alive again. He insists that - similar to the handling of children's feelings of loss when in hospital - poor handling of the experience may have severe consequences. It may lead to 'pathological mourning', which, in adulthood, may contribute to the development of a psychotic depressive illness. Healthy mourning in adults, as in children, goes through the earlier mentioned three stages of 'protest', 'despair' and 'detachment' (with a period of numbness preceding these stages in adults). The security of the bond with the 'lost 'person as well as the understanding of the child's reactions are vital. Bowlby says 'nothing but confusion and pathology results when the news of the death is withheld or glossed over (even in the case of suicide). Expression of emotion, yearning, even anger must be encouraged, crying not even implicitly discouraged, sorrow must be shared between the survivors'.

The child's feelings of guilt–anger against the surviving parent – almost invariably present in a case of suicide, or where parent relationship was poor – must be voiced and discussed. The persistence of memories and even vivid images of the dead person must be expected. Bowlby is convinced that there is no fundamental difference between children's and adults' reactions to loss and death and he quotes Darwin (1877), who traces much of the adults' expression in times of grief to the crying of an infant: 'In all cases of distress our brains tend through long habit to send an order to certain muscles to contract, as if we were still infants on the point of screaming out'. Children's common fears after the experience of death of a parent are:

(1) They themselves, or the surviving parent, might die.
(2) They might have caused the death.
(3) They will be reunited with the loved person either by death or by the dead person's return to life; this idea may often be triggered off by the sick parent being taken to the hospital before dying having said 'I shall soon be back'.

One of the consequences of pathological mourning is that grief may be too intense or too prolonged, based on anxious and insecure attachment. Fugue states, partly provoked by an anxious search for the lost person, may occur and pathological insistency on self-sufficiency with repression of the death, and severe depression are common. Despite some equivocal research findings, depression seems to occur more often after the loss of a parent before the eleventh birthday. In Brown *et al.*'s (1977) famous London study of 558 women, 42.5% of the 40 depressed women had lost their mother before the eleventh birthday, while of the 418 who lived with mother throughout their youth, only 14% became depressed.

Loss of father may occur not only through death but also through divorce. Wallerstein *et al.* (1975) studied 34 children immediately after the divorce and 1 year later. Despite the fact that these children remained with mother in familiar surroundings, the youngest group, $2\frac{1}{2}$–$3\frac{1}{2}$ years old, showed typical reactions: regression in toilet training, crying, increased fearfulness, sleep problems, temper tantrums, etc.; but the adverse effects subsided after 1 year, provided substitute care-taking was good and there was no continuance of the discord which had led to the divorce. The children were left only with an increased need of comfort from any adults. In the $3\frac{3}{4}$–$4\frac{3}{4}$-year-olds, regression was evident only in half of the cases immediately after the divorce, but 1 year later all these children seemed bewildered as though their concept of the dependability of human relationships was shaken forever. They blamed themselves for the loss, very similar to the reaction of children who lose a parent through death. Mothers in these cases had often been frantically preoccupied with adjusting to the new situation and had been less available to the children.

Of the 5–6-year-olds only a few showed signs of depression and poor peer relationships after a year had passed. In these cases divorce had been preceded by stormy relationships between the parents and divorce had solved some of the family problems. Divorce seems particularly difficult for girls when father leaves the family. Not only developmental physicians must take seriously the loss of a parent for the child, especially if it is before the age of 11 years. All care-givers – including teachers and relations who see children – must be aware of the possible consequences of such a loss.

Bowlby's advice about the handling of mourning as described above may bring the child relief, prevent maladjustment and even avoid gross disorders in later life – it should help towards healthy 'detachment' and the establishment of new ties to new people to replace the lost figure.

# Chapter 5

# WHO AM I? THE ESTABLISHMENT OF IDENTITY

## (A) GENDER IDENTITY

A preschool child is not usually brought to a clinic with the explicit problem of confusion about sexual identity. Boys with conspicuously effeminate behaviour (and what is considered 'effeminate' varies considerably according to the social background) are sometimes investigated, while girls who behave unusually tomboyishly are almost always tolerated within the family, with the idea that they will 'grow out of it'. However, almost all of the male transexualists who desire to become females (and females who desire to become males) are firmly convinced that their deviance was clear to them before entering kindergarten. Parents were insensitive to the abnormality for a long while; only now – partly as a consequence of media interest in the condition – are they more aware of possible severe deviations. At what time do children recognize sex differences? At what time do they normally acquire the desire to play the feminine or masculine role which our culture assigns to them? At what time is their sexual orientation firmly established and how does so-called masculinity and femininity develop?

There are three main theories to explain the development of appropriate, socially approved, sex-typed behaviour and heterosexual choice. Firstly, psychoanalysis claims that people are basically bisexual. Deviant sexual patterns such as homosexuality or fetishism are said to be normal in childhood and their persistence into adult life, in the face of social disapproval, is said to be due to regression or fixation at the early childhood level. Treatment consists in attempting to solve the problem which caused the regression. The second theory, the social learning theory, claims that socially approved masculinity and femininity (and heterosexual choice in adulthood) are the result of learning through reward and punishment, observation and imitation. This theory simply explains 'abnormal' sexual behaviour in adult life as being learned from deviant models in childhood.

Into this framework fits the theory formulated by the American workers Money *et al.* (1957) who talk about 'psychosexual neutrality' at birth. They formed their theories on the basis of observation of a large number of cases where the biological sex and the sex of rearing were different, i.e. biological males were brought up as females and vice versa. These workers found that, almost universally, the individuals chose to remain in the sex role in which they were reared even if in adolescence it became clear that their biological sex was different. Money and his co-workers believe that social influence is so important that change in the sex role becomes aversive to the subject. They spell out the pressures which, from early childhood onwards, are exerted on the child to conform to the masculine or feminine image.

The third theory, also fitting in with Money's observations, is cognitive developmental: it claims that sexual identity is established by the child due to its need to preserve a stable, positive self-image. This becomes stable when the child realizes the stability of objects in general, which according to Kohlberg (1969) occurs after 6 - years the same time as children learn the principle of conservation. Gesell reported in 1940 that two-thirds to three-quarters of all

3-year-olds answered correctly the question: 'Are you a girl or a boy?', while most 2½-year-olds did not.

However, knowing that he or she is a boy or a girl does not mean that the child can recognize another child's sex. At 4 years the child still decides on the basis of hairstyle, etc. and children under 5 years of age believe that a boy will become a girl by growing his hair and wearing a skirt. (They also believe that a cat can become a dog.) By 6 years they know that their sex cannot be changed, that gender is permanent and not subject to spontaneous and wilful change, although an understanding that gender is determined on the basis of genitals instead of on the basis of behaviour (such as preference for certain toys, which is already different for boys and girls at 13 months) does not develop until 7–9 years, according to McConaghy (1979).

Final awareness that it is the genital difference which is the dominant characteristic, differentiating boys from girls, is not common before 11 years of age. Once the certainty of gender has been established, the child will imitate and appreciate those behaviour patterns which are consistent with its own gender and from the knowledge 'I am a male' (or a female) develops the need to behave in a masculine or feminine fashion. An investigation carried out in 1947, based on interviews with children, confirmed that one half of them thought that girls had had a penis which they lost, but not all of those who thought so seemed to be perturbed by this idea. However, this investigation is a partial confirmation of the psychoanalytical postulate about children's fantasies about sex and castration.

## (B) HUMAN DIMORPHISM AND SIBLING RIVALRY

There are those who altogether disbelieve that sex-appropriate behaviour is entirely learned and that this learning occurs in early childhood. They say that sex-appropriate behaviour is the unfolding of a biologically laid down pattern which includes not only direct sexual activities but lifestyles, which are widely different for males and females. Cultural and social pressures act upon an organism which already has certain predispositions and propensities. Biology and culture are therefore aspects of a continued process of interaction. This theory is advocated by Hutt (1972); she stresses the fact that the developmental time-table is different for males and females throughout life: females develop faster in the early stages and a gradual decline in some aspects of mental function seems to set in earlier in females. Male deaths in the first year of life are 25% more than female deaths in all cultures. Girl babies not only sit up, walk and above all, talk 2-6 weeks earlier than boys, they retain their advantage in most aspects of the language area (except for vocabulary) until adult life.

Moreover, it is difficult to explain, on the basis of social learning theory, the greater spelling ability of girls and the equally greater ability of boys to cope with spatial problems: clearly these skills were not specially modelled by the same-sex parent and imitated by the child. Also, the difference in verbal ability between boys and girls declines during adolescence, just in the very period when growing identification with the same-sex parent ought to increase it. Goodenough in 1931 reported that anger is shown at 7 months of age in boys and not by girls.

The advantage in the language area may, indeed, be biologically useful for girls, since it facilitates person-to-person communication and contributes to the forging of personal social relationships. Female babies *hear* better, while male babies *see* better, and the differing preference for one or the other sensory channel is manifest even in later life, when (according to Kinsey *et al.* (1948)) men are more sexually aroused by visual erotic stimuli and women by touch. Hutt (1972) says: 'the sensitivity, first evident in the cradle, is amply exploited by the stripteaser and pornographer'. (The experimental basis for the greater sensitivity of boy babies to visual stimuli and girl babies for auditory stimuli has been challenged by some investigators in recent years; see Birns (1977).)

Some of the striking differences between boys and girls during the preschool years might be the direct result of the slower general rate of maturation of boys: for instance, so-called congenital reading retardation is almost five times as common in boys as girls, perhaps due to their slower maturation in the language area.

Stammering is four times as common in boys. In child-guidance clinics, twice as many boys as girls are seen for conduct disorder, since immature boys, confronted with demands which require maturity, may be unable to cope and therefore react with behaviour problems. Autism with its important language deficit is also four times more common in boys.

Moreover, differences in the strength and kind of aggression between boys and girls is clearly shown in preschool age. At 3 years the difference has been noted in nursery schools, boys having more aggressive contacts with peers than girls have, and this difference is shown to exist in six cultures, studied by the Whitings (1975). In the West it may already be influenced by social factors, approval or disapproval by adults. In the so-called 'permissive doll play', where a child sitting in front of a doll's house is encouraged to act out its fantasies and ideas about father, mother, siblings etc., boys show aggression in their play which is often destructive and hurtful, while girls show predominantly verbal aggression in play, i.e. the so-called 'prosocial aggression' – punishment meted out for misbehaviour. The same difference is shown when boys and girls are tested with a similar test at age 12.

The clinician will have to be aware of the normal jealousies between boys and girl children at this stage when the young boy, jealous of the comparative maturity of his little sister, may be seriously threatened in his self-esteem and his feelings of his own worth. On the other hand, the girl, jealous of the brother's more assertive and aggressive personality, may reject her tendency to gentleness and 'femininity', emulate a boyish stance and behaviour (described in psychoanalytic terms as 'penis envy'). Exceptionally severe rivalries between opposite-sex siblings leads to maladjustment in adult life in the field of educational and occupational ambition and in marital and parental behaviour. Developmental paediatricians may help normal development by their sensitivity and awareness of incipient dangers.

Large-scale researches by Sears *et al.* (1957), who investigated the parents' attitudes about what constitutes 'masculinity' and 'femininity', did not find any significant correlation with the children's actual behaviour. Nor did the parents' expectation of what they considered appropriate sex behaviour show any correlation with the children's attitudes.

Only a few grossly abnormal features were significantly correlated in Sears' data: father's sexual anxieties as well as mother's punitiveness, a great amount of physical punishment by either parent and severe weaning and toilet-training procedures all seemed to some extent to contribute to feminization in both sexes.

Families where fathers were absent did not contain a significantly greater number of boys with non-masculine orientation. Father's absence, however, in some cases retarded the expression of masculinity. There was also no evidence for the importance of separation from the same-sex parent for the later sexual orientation of the child. Death of fathers does *not* result in feminization of boys.

In the absence of environmental features, which are clearly causative in atypical sexual orientation of children, it seems more and more likely that, indeed, as Hutt (1972) asserted, there is a hitherto unknown biological factor which encourages male (or female) children to refuse and reject the lifestyles assigned to them in our culture. Many transexuals insist, even in the face of great difficulties, on 'sex change' operations. Some cultures have developed institutions designed to accommodate people with such atypical sex attitude. For instance, in some Red Indian cultures there exist ways to allow and even to encourage boys to wear female dress. They can opt out of the ceremonies designed to show off masculinity and, in a number of such cultures, these 'female' men have great prestige and act as advisers in communal conflicts.

Female cross-gender cases are fewer and less studied because of the greater frequency with which 'tomboyish' girls change their behaviour at puberty. On the other hand, there are a number of interesting longitudinal studies in which 'feminine' boys are followed up and treated at age 4-10, reported by Green (1977). All the children are anatomically normal and their economic, social and ethnic background is varied. The parents are seen and the children are investigated by various tests, and on the basis of this - still incomplete - study, the authors enumerate various possible aetiological factors for 'femininity' in boys:

(1) An innate dislike of rough-and-tumble play and aggressive activities.
(2) Unusual physical beauty, causing those around him to treat the boy as a girl.
(3) Family encouragement of cross-dressing and unmasculine behaviour.
(4) Maternal over-protection and unavailability of male playmates during the first years of socialization.
(5) Absence of a male model during the first years or rejection by the father.

(Green suggests early psychiatric treatment, and I will discuss this in a later chapter.) The central and most important focus in a treatment plan is the establishment of a new father-son relationship, while other therapists emphasize the need for changing mothers' attitudes; mothers – owing to their unconscious dislike of men – may subtly encourage their sons' femininity (Newman 1977).

## (C) ROLE OF THE FATHER

What *is* the role of the father in the nuclear family of Western society? In psychological as well as in psycho-analytic theory the infant–mother relationship has always been considered unique, the prototype of all later loving relationships. In psychoanalysis father's importance be-comes paramount for the boy only in later preschool years, described as the 'oedipal' phase, when the boy strives to identify with the father as a result of fears that his intimate attachment to his mother might be punished.

Is there any evidence supporting the assumption that, therefore, the absence of a father prevents the smooth accomplishment of the process of gender orientation? Will too close a relationship to mother lead to homosexuality? The evidence is not convincing, and empirical results do not support the theory that identification with the father-figure is the only source of masculine sex orientation in later life. The child takes as a model not only the like-sex parent, but it learns sex typing from other sources – often from other children. Even if reared in sexually atypical households, for instance by lesbian couples, boys do not generally develop abnormally.

According to Kinsey *et al.* (1948) 4% of men are exclu-sively homosexual. Kallman (1952) found 100% concord-ance in monozygotic twins and only 30% concordance in dizygotic twins and believes that a constitutional factor is involved. However, newer twin studies have not found the same results. Mischel (1970) quotes a study by Greenskin carried out in 1966, in which postpubertal boys taking sodium amytal medication answered carefully structured questions about homosexual encounters. No differences were found between those boys where father was absent from the home and those where father was present. Older children clearly found masculine models outside the house if no father-figure lived at home.

Boys between 13 and 15 who have experience of mutual masturbation do not consider themselves to be homosexual. Between 15 and 16 mutual masturbation begins to be recognized as homosexual behaviour and tends to evoke shame and guilt. After this the homosexual boy adjusts to his condition. Homosexual seduction during adolescence does not necessarily cause homosexuality, unless later reinforcing factors strengthen the homosexual trend. However, a great proportion of homosexuals describe themselves as having been girl-like during childhood. In one study of such 'feminine' boys, 15 out of 27 are now atypical adults. However, investigations of boys who have grown up without a father in the home indicate that although they are not homosexual, heterosexual relationships in adulthood are more difficult for them than for those reared in 'normal' families. They are not feminine, but often seem to have to prove their masculinity and therefore find stable heterosexual relationships hard to maintain.

The Whitings (1975) assert that societies with exclusive mother–son sleeping arrangements have elaborate male initiation rites, as if to psychologically brainwash the child and turn his previous feminine identity forcefully towards the masculine role. Some present writers believe that the 'gang', with its preoccupation with toughness, plays a similar role for the lower-class urban boy who is brought up in a preponderantly matriarchal household.

## (D) GROUP FORMATION AND FRIENDSHIPS

While research into the role of the father, which had been neglected owing to the belief of the paramount influence of the mother-infant relationship, has been revived, research into the function of children's groups has also recently aroused interest under the influence of sociologists, ethologists and ecologists. Susan Isaacs (1933) still says: 'The child is a naive egoist – other children are mainly rivals for the love and approval of adults.' However, we now know that children's groupings have an immense influence on development. Harlow's (1974) investigations a few years ago already served to strengthen the conviction of the importance of the peer group: they demonstrated that the loss of playmates is even more devastating for the small rhesus monkey than the absence of mother. Rhesus monkeys deprived of playmates between 6 and 12 months not only failed to establish normal behaviour when returned to their group, they were also sexually deviant and poor parents.

Bowlby (1979) has noted the change in attachment behaviour at the beginning of the fourth year, which clearly is linked to the beginning of the child's establishing ties to its peers.

There is a pattern of intersex communication in children of Western society: in play groups, nurseries and parks, where children get together, there is little evidence of sex preference in 2-year-olds. But by 3–4 years there are changes in both the size of the groups and their sex distribution. By 2 years, toddlers form groups in twosomes – there are hardly ever groups of three or more (see Figure 6). Contrastingly, by 4 years there are larger groupings and they become concerned with belonging: the children begin to choose other children of the same sex and of the same set as friends and playmates. The 'in' and 'out' ritual and the establishment of deviancy begins. By 11 years the sex segregation has become almost total (Figure 9). Boys are determined to exclude girls and girls to exclude boys. A recent experiment carried out by Serbin *et al.* (1977), with 4-year-olds, aimed at encouraging boys and girls to share their games, rewarding cross-sex play pattern. Serbin was

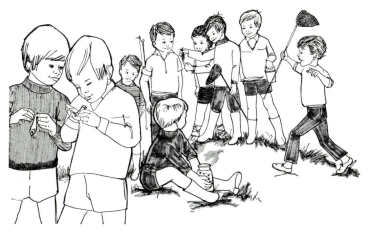

Figure 9    Typical boy nursery group [reproduced from
*Males and Females* (Hutt, 1972), Penguin Books]

successful as long as the experiment lasted, but the former
pattern of strict sex segregation was re-established as soon
as the encouragement was withdrawn. The segregation is
apparently seen between the ages of 5 and 11 in primitive
cultures and it exists in primates. Boys' groups tend to
band together in rebellious attitudes – if not for delinquent
acts then for pranks and resistance to adults. Girls tend to
form a network of intimate relationships, often two by two
linked to other pairs.

Bernal (1974) quotes Kohlberg (1969), who denies that
security and contact comfort are the main factors in the
development of social behaviour. After all, the rhesus monkeys with surrogate mothers lacking playmates have 'secure' physical contacts but they are not social. Kohlberg
believes that in humans there is an intrinsic motivation to
engage in social interaction. He doubts that the relationship with mother is more important for the development
of social bonds than, for example, the relationship with
siblings.

Experiences with peer groups help the child to develop

both an awareness of social reality and a sense of identity. The child's concept of himself develops in a social nexus, in which the peer group is an important agent. Hartup (1970) says the group is an agent of social control in maintaining and changing the behaviour of the individual. It is a source of social norms. There are definite stages in the development of friendship and of play patterns. The infant of 1 year explores another baby only as a physical object, without engaging it in play. At $2\frac{1}{2}$ years, children begin to have some sort of social interaction; they clearly distinguish inanimate objects from children, realizing that another child can both initiate social behaviour and respond to it. They no longer play solitary, independent games but engage in 'parallel activity', playing with toys the other children play with, but *along* rather than *with* the other child.

Piaget has described the 'collective monologue' at this stage in play groups when children prattle and put questions while playing, but never expect an answer and never answer other children's questions; they are largely unaware of others. Then follows the 'associative' play, including borrowing and loaning of play materials; fluctuating altruistic behaviour and sympathy begin to develop, and also competition and rivalry, but there are as yet no organized games. At $3\frac{1}{2}$ years the incidence of complex interchange with other children equals or exceeds the incidence of such interaction by the same children with adults.

Between $3\frac{1}{2}$ and 5 years, children say they have friends. However, friendship does not mean more than having momentary playmates who may change any time. There is no mutuality and no permanence in these friendships (Rubin 1980). Awareness of permanence of the relationship is found only after 6 years. The friend does things for you, he does things that please you, but there is still no reciprocity. This, according to Piaget (1965), is not in the child's repertoire before the age of 7 years.

However, Waldrop and Halverson (1976) conclude from

a longitudinal study that children who at age 2½ were 'friendly involved' with their peers and able to cope with aggressive children of their own age were likely, when aged 7½, to be 'socially at ease'. They are the ones who decide with whom they want to play. Sociability at age 2½ was thus positively related to sociability 5 years later.

## (E) WORKING MOTHERS AND THE RISKS OF DAY CARE

All investigations of group influence emphasize that the exclusive interest in maternal attachment in previous studies has missed one more essential fact, vital to human social development: the child's wider surroundings, the social network in which the family is involved, plays so important a part that it must not be disregarded. This has been shown in the Swansea team's (Hall and Stacey, 1979) research on hospitalized children, quoted earlier, where the separation from the familiar surroundings of the home was shown to be at least as causative of the child's distress in hospital as was the separation from mother. In this light, the question of the usefulness and risks of toddlers' play groups and child-minding arrangements must be reconsidered.

Swedish researchers, reported by Bronfenbrenner (1979), have pointed out that in the 'natural' – mostly non-urban – family setting, apart from mother, there are neighbours, relations and friends who sometimes act as care-takers and the child can experiment with all sorts of non-play material such as mother's possessions and her plants and kitchen equipment; the child has varied opportunities for exploration and learning. One of the English investigators (Moore 1972) has found that boys who had diffuse mothering with frequent substitute care before the child's fourth birthday come to care less for the approval of adults and more for that of their peers. They tend to become more active, assertive and independent. On the other hand, boys who had been fully in care of their mother until school age tend to internalize adult standards of behaviour and learn self-control, but this attitude tends to persist into adolescence and leads to the inhibition of assertive behaviour with detrimental consequences. However, in inner-city life substitute care for children, even before 18 months, is the usual and unavoidable consequence either of economic necessity or the need for independence of young mothers who do not want exclusive child-care responsibilities.

These children are unavoidably cared for not by the parents in a home such as described by the Swedish researchers, but by complete strangers who, in their turn, have neither relations nor neighbours to help in the care-taking. Rutter (1981) has summarized what is now known about the usefulness and risks of day care for young children whose own parents and own homes are not available to them, except after the parents come home from work. He tried to evaluate the advantages and disadvantages of all sorts of arrangements for day care of the young child.

Clearly, the quality of the early care provided at home, as well as the quality of the substitute care, are vital factors. The adequacy of substitute arrangements vary to a terrifying extent and the innumerable new researches which try to pinpoint the disadvantages and advantages of day-care facilities are not conclusive, according to Rutter. Nevertheless he is sure that day care even for small children is not fundamentally detrimental to the process of bonding. The baby continues his attachment to mother at home while in day care, in contrast to the situation in full residential care. It cannot be said that mother's working outside the home necessarily disrupts the attachment process essential for the child's further development provided that she and father have time and enjoyment in playing with the child (Figure 10). Young children in day care often develop a secondary attachment to one of the care-takers,

*Who am I? The establishment of identity*

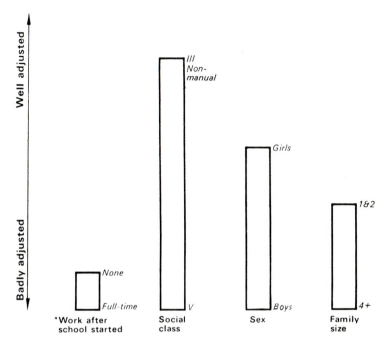

*There was no effect of the mother working *before* school
started upon the children's social adjustment

Figure 10   Relation between mother's working and children's social adjustment in school [reproduced with permission from *From Birth to Seven* (Davie Butler and Goldstein, 1972), p. 46, Longman]

and it is important that these do not change too often and that the child is not forced to cope with separation from this secondary figure of attachment too often or too early.

In the older child, between 3 and 5 years, the advantages of play groups, day-care centres or extended foster families are substantial: they teach the child to get along with peers, thus preparing him for experiences which will challenge him in school. The points emerging from Rutter's (1981) review are: firstly, the need for a high staff–child ratio in play groups for young children; secondly, care must include play, conversation and emotional comfort as well as super-vision of physical needs; thirdly, first-born and boys are somewhat more vulnerable to the experience of separation from home; and fourthly, a separation from home is prob-ably most detrimental between 7 and 18 months when bonds are being formed and the growth of fear is maximal.

In this chapter I have tried to trace the beginning of the establishment of personal and social identity in the young child, in the period between babyhood and the elementary school years. The child starts this period confined to the world of his own family, where interactions happen within the 'dyadic' systems of mother–infant or infant–sibling relationships. When the child enters school, on the other hand, he is expected to have learned to co-operate with strangers, children and adults. In 1902 Baldwin, quoted by Cairn *et al.* (1980), said: 'The development of the child's personality cannot go on at all without the constant mod-ification of his sense of himself by suggestion from others.' Children learn from others, taking an active role in social-izing each other long before elementary school. When en-tering school the child is expected to know what and who he or she is. Boy or girl, dependent or independent, fearful or courageous, he or she is expected to behave accordingly. The clinician's role in this development is to help parents and children to handle incipient deviances and to prevent social isolation.

# Chapter 6

---

# THE MIDDLE SCHOOL YEARS

---

## (A) THE LEARNING OF MORAL JUDGEMENT

It is during the school years that the child acquires the value system of Western culture and learns to act in accordance with society's moral code, even on occasions when there is no external authority to threaten punishment for digression. There is – as already shown – a period during the child's first year when obedience to mother's commands comes almost unquestionably, and there is the toddler stage where disobedience is a common pattern, assertion against parental wishes becoming for the child a symbol and a manifestation of beginning independence. But what is the route by which the child learns to distinguish between 'good' and 'bad', between what is permitted and what is forbidden by society and culture, and how does he learn to act accordingly, even when there is nobody present to tell him? How does he learn to submit to rules which run counter to his wishes? Why does he comply with society's demands, that he should attend school and submit to the school's discipline, while he would prefer to play in the street? How does he acquire emotions such as feelings of guilt or shame after transgression? How does he learn to be helpful and sympathetic – how does he acquire the so-called 'prosocial' attitudes?

There are (Hoffman 1970) three fundamental theories about children's socialization: there is the theory of 'original sin', modified by Freud in whose theories the pleasure-seeking Id has to be restrained and socialized during development; there is Rousseau's assertion of the total innocence of childhood with its innate altruism, destroyed or threatened by society; and there is the theory of a tabula rasa, adopted by learning theory, which assumes that all judgements about how to behave are learned by reward and punishment, modelling and imitation. Piaget (1965) who devoted much of his researches to the question of how moral judgement is being learned, says 'the essence of morality includes both respect for the rules of social order, and a sense of justice, i.e. concern for reciprocity and equality among individuals'.

The methods by which Piaget studied the growth of moral judgement were highly original: he observed children's play and he systematically questioned children of all ages: which of two actions is more 'wrong' and why? Which of two judgements is more appropriate? Why do the children think so? The child in preschool and early school years is in Piaget's terms a 'moral realist'. He believes in 'immanent justice'; he is convinced that violation of norms is inevitably followed by accident and misfortune willed by God, or caused by inanimate objects. Rules are, according to the child, sacred; they have been there forever; they are unalterable, rigid; obedience is obligatory.

Change from 'heteronomy' towards the second stage, described as 'autonomous morality', depends on maturation. It is possible only in interaction with peers and the parents, who teach the child to take on the 'role of the other'. In this way he comes to realize that the rights of the other are the same as those he claims for himself, i.e. he learns 'reciprocity' in the moral area in the same way as he has to learn reciprocity in other areas: the moon does not accompany only himself when he walks, but equally accompanies a child going in the opposite direction; he, Peter, not only has a brother called Paul, but Paul equally has a brother called Peter, etc. When the child has learned reciprocity, rules are no longer regarded as unchangeable and ordained for ever by external forces, but they are seen as established and maintained by agreement among those who abide by them and are subject to modification by consent which is binding on each of the partners.

He learns to appreciate that actions are not 'good' or 'bad' according to the dictum of external authority or according to the consequences, but that their moral value depends on the intention of the perpetrator of the act. At what age the child will grasp the concept of justice in the sense that Western society uses it depends on his cognitive maturation, as well as on the opportunities he is given for experiences in interaction with others. According to Piaget (1965) it occurs in the middle of the school years, roughly at the transition to secondary school.

Learning theorists also believe that experience with equals and verbal interaction with parents is the essential condition for the eventual acquisition of moral rules, even in the absence of reward and punishment, while during preschool and in early school years, reward and punishment is the main method to teach a child to conform. Learning theorists stress the importance of imitation of models. They deny that there is any fundamental difference between the concepts of imitation and identification, the term in which the internalization of moral rules is couched in analytical theory.

Analysts believe in the emergence of the 'conscience', the internalization of moral demands, at 5–6 years: the child at first feels hostile to the parents, because by threats of punishment or abandonment they frustrate his wishes for immediate gratification. Nevertheless the child finally adopts the parental commands by 'anaclitic identification', erecting defences against any impulse to contravene parental demands. To the degree to which parents' discipline arouses anxiety over loss of love (or of castration) the child strives to incorporate the parents – including their moral standards. He allays his anxieties by this internalization of the parents' moral values – internalized parents can no longer abandon him. The child then feels anxiety at his antisocial impulses and represses them, even in the absence of external threat; guilt feelings follow transgression.

However, research shows that identification – the internalization of parental standards – is not a unitary process and that children identify often, not with the parents, but with people outside the home. They learn some of their morals from parents and some from peers. Moreover, it is not only the threatening aspect of the parent but it is their loving aspect which is also incorporated and forms the conscience (the superego).

## (B) PARENTAL REARING SYSTEMS

Social learning theory sees the child's fears of withdrawal of love by the parents as one of the main agents by which the child learns conformity to social rules. Peer relationship is seen as another important agent in teaching moral judgement. Hoffman (1970) stresses the influence of the parents' teaching methods: these are seen either as 'power assertive' or non-assertive. All studies show that fundamentally there are very different consequences of these two methods of handling children's transgressions of social rules. There was a high correlation between 'power assertive' child-rearing patterns and *weak* subsequent moral development. (These studies were almost all concerned with middle-class American children.) Power assertion by the parent resulted in expressions of rage, frustrating the child's need for autonomy; it fostered the image of the parent and authority as arbitrary and provided the child with a model for discharging anger. The consequence is *not* the internalization of the rules but a tendency to avoid the power-assertive agent.

Among the non-power-assertive methods the sheer threat of withdrawal of love was also shown to be ineffective, except that it contributed to inhibition of anger. It provoked anxiety about transgression but did not induce internalization of moral rules. On the other hand, 'induction' has been shown to contribute to the suppression of antisocial impulses. Induction is also a non-assertive method; it consists of explanations of demands in terms the child can understand, of an appeal to the child's innate tendency to feel sympathy, and it expounds the harm transgression does to others.

In summary, Hoffman concludes that moral development is a complex multifaceted phenomenon to which several different processes contribute: in the very young child specific acts will be labelled as 'good' or 'bad' if followed by immediate contingent reward or punishment. With further development the child learns, by imitation or identification with authority figures, the rules of behaviour, accepted in his environment. Finally, the child, with the help of explanation or by participation in decision-making or by role-playing adult roles, is mature enough to re-evaluate the world of authority, learn to inhibit impulses and acquire consideration of others' rights. He will then (one hopes) no longer comply for fear of punishment and loss of love but anxiety, originally associated with threats, will become associated with the antisocial impulse itself, so that such urges are suppressed even in the absence of authority and will result in feelings of guilt.

However, it has been shown by experimental evidence that the recognition of moral values, and even the strength of guilt feelings and shame after transgression are not highly correlated with behaviour. Delinquents may act antisocially despite the strength of guilt feelings afterwards.

Resistance to antisocial impulses is highly dependent on the specific situation in which they arise.

Hartshorne and May's famous study (1928) using 11 000 children aged 11–16 years, who were given the opportunity to cheat or to lie (without noticing that they were observed), showed that 'dishonest' children in one situation behaved 'honestly' in another one. Although recent studies of Hartshorne and May's statistics have modified their conclusions somewhat, their dictum, which states that 'honest' is not a unitary trait of character and personality, has not been refuted. Insight into the moral value of an act or guilt feelings at transgression are not good predictors of behaviour.

## (C) THE SCHOOL AS A SOCIAL INSTITUTION

On the other hand, interaction with peers does tend to teach a sense of mutuality at school age and this leads to modification of impulsive antisocial behaviour. Equality of rights is part of school life: 'It's my turn. . . '. 'Now it's your turn . . .' is one of the ways leading towards the learning of reciprocity. Schools are clearly not solely the transmitters of information and educational skills; they are powerful institutions for socialization, for moulding children's behaviour and attitudes. Research into the specific methods by which they achieve this has hitherto been neglected by psychological theorists. Rutter's (1976b) research team estimated that children spend 15 000 hours of their lives in school, and although a preponderance of children which are seen in clinical practice are schoolchildren, little is known about what this institution can and cannot do. This is partly due to methodological problems: how does one separate the influence of school on the child from home influence? How far are the differences in behavioural patterns between children in different schools due to differences in the background from which they came?

# The middle school years

Despite these problems – and after years of painstaking research work – Rutter's team published findings about school influence which are most revealing and far too little known: parents were always anxious to get their child allotted to the 'right' school, even when the choice was only between different secondary schools with similar curriculums. Nevertheless, it was until recently accepted as an undisputed fact (mostly on the basis of evidence collected in America) that home influences far outweigh those of the school – even though it was known, for instance, that in one English county some Comprehensive schools achieved 6% and others 32% examination successes and equally widely divergent rates of successes were obtained in Grammar schools (which took 15% of the most academically advanced children). Some schools obtained 26%, others 78% successes. It is mainly the hope to give their children a chance for educational success which made parents anxious about the choice of secondary school.

However, school influences not only examination results: it is a potent factor in a child's social development. Rutter's research team (Rutter *et al.* 1979) had the unique advantage of having at their disposal a body of measurements relating to 1400 children, their personalities, social backgrounds, and intellectual level before their entrance to those secondary schools which the team investigated. The researchers therefore were able to judge how far the successes which the schools obtained were due solely to the choice of children they took from the primary schools. Was there a change for better or worse after entrance into secondary school? Which were the secondary schools that effected changes in the children for the better and which were the ones where school influence led to a deterioration in socialization?

One well-known investigation (Power *et al.* 1967) found huge differences in delinquency rates between different secondary schools serving the same London borough.

Social development

Annual average delinquency rates varied from 1 to 19%. Their rates stayed the same over 6 years. Another recent study of schools in an outer London suburb, of rather different social characteristics, showed similar variation. (This study included referrals to child-guidance clinics and found high delinquency rates to go hand in hand with high referrals to CGC for emotional disorders.) Rutter's research focusses on the children's behaviour in school, the rate of non-attendance, the examination successes and the rates of delinquency in 12 secondary schools attended by a particularly disadvantaged population. Again, very large variations were found between different schools (in boys' schools the delinquency rate varied from 0–31%). The behavioural deviancy rate (judged from teachers' questionnaires) ranged from 0–48% and reading difficulties from 6–26%. Were these variations merely reflections of differences between the schools in the proportion of difficult children they admitted? This was the first question and the answer was 'no'. The difference between schools in the intake of children aged 11 years did not explain the difference between them when the children were aged 14. The schools with the most promising intake were not necessarily those with the best outcome.

Furthermore, schools with similar intakes sometimes had very different findings at age 14. For instance, one school which had 30% children with behaviour difficulty at age 10 had only 9.2% at age 14, while another with 34% at age 10 had 48% at age 14. The findings suggested that some schools were able to exert a positive and beneficial influence on their pupils and protected them to some extent from difficulties.

What were the reasons for the discrepancies between schools? Why were the outcomes adverse in some while others did well by the pupils, even if they had arrived at age 10 equally difficult or equally promising? Rutter's researchers were positive that age of school building, ability streaming, teacher–pupil ratio, etc. were not significant factors contributing to high or low delinquency rates, to poor or good behaviour, to examination results, or to erratic school attendance.

The features which, on the other hand, correlated with good outcomes in terms of the areas on which the study focussed were: emphasis on academic progress (including the setting and checking of homework), planning of the curriculum, use of library facilities, punctuality by the teacher and good use of teaching time, etc. While there was no correlation between outcome and severity of punishment, there was a correlation between outcome and the amount of reward and praise given. Moreover, the outcome was good in those schools which gave children responsibilities, where there were flowers in the windows and clean corridors, where teachers were available for private discussions and advice to the children and where the teachers in their turn felt supervised and guided by the senior staff. The authors summarize their findings, stating that:

'Because we had information on what the children were like before they entered secondary school, we knew that the difference in school attendance, in behaviour and attainment as well as the rates of delinquency had arisen as a result of changes in children's performance after secondary transfer. Their behaviour and attainments, while at secondary school, were not just a continuation of patterns already established at an earlier age. Instead it seemed that children's experience during their years of secondary school had played a part in shaping their development and these changes were systematically related to measures characteristic of the schools they attended. This increased the likelihood that the link with the school was indeed the result of causal processes.'

Thus, children's behaviour and attitudes are shaped and influenced by their experience at school and in particular by the quality of the school as a social institution. The mechanisms by which the norms for the school as a social institution are established are: teacher's expectations, the model they provide, and the feedback the child receives on what is acceptable performance at his school. The conditions which make for acceptance by the pupils of these norms are: staff concern for the children, high expectation by the teachers, shared activities among pupils and staff and shared responsibilities and experience of success. The authors' conclusion is that even in a disadvantaged area, schools can be a force for the good.

## (D) THE ACQUISITION OF SOCIAL SKILLS

The child's time in school is not only spent in the classroom. School age is the primary period in which the child begins to perceive the consequences of success and failure and initiates the response patterns which will influence his eventual attitude to work: school years are formative for the acquisition of social skills and the ability to exercise interpersonal control (Weinstein 1969). Very few data are available to tell us how people learn to exercise control over others and to acquire 'interpersonal competence' so important for future success. In order to learn how to get other people to act in the way you want them to, you need empathy and the understanding of reciprocity – principles learned in the middle-school years. Even 3-year-old children show sympathy: they elicit the help of adults when they see another child being hurt. But more is needed for true empathy. It includes 'projective role taking', the ability to understand how someone else would feel and act in a particular situation. This in turn depends on the similarity between one's own experience and that of others. There is greater empathy within than across social and ethnic categories and school groups form on the basis of similarity. Racial awareness begins in nurseries at the age of

4 years; it increases with age until pre-adolescence and may then decline.

However, common experience even within different social and ethnic backgrounds occurs in school, and the child learns – to some extent – how different categories of people feel: this is invaluable and is one of the reasons for establishing mixed-class and inter-racial schools.

Middle childhood is a period of increasingly explicit and rigid conformity to social norms; conformity increases until adolescence, when the youth begins to question and reassess prejudices and social rules.

## (E) LEARNING CONTROL OF AGGRESSION AND THE INFLUENCE OF THE MASS MEDIA

Moreover, and surprisingly, aggression is less violent in middle school years than in early childhood (Table 3). Perhaps this is so because the child in school learns to cope with frustration and anger by non-violent methods, or perhaps because of his increasing ability to use fantasy as a means to express internally feelings and wishes, including hostile ones. The need to act out directly by aggression is thereby diminished. The tendency to react to frustration and pain with aggressive acts is more pronounced in some children than in others – almost certainly on a genetic basis, according to Shaffer *et al.* (1980). It is not unlikely that a long Y chromosome is the cause, since the tendency to aggression is stronger in males than females even in non-Western cultures (and equally in non-human primates). Boys are four times more likely than girls to develop conduct disorders. Fire setting at the ages of 6–8 years is exclusively done by boys, and it is probable that the magic properties boys see in fire expresses their aggressive feelings about important adults, congruent with analytical theories that fire is symbolically related to male sexuality.

Aggressive and assertive behaviour is one of the few

Table 3  Some developmental aspects of violence

| Age | Type | Object | Aim | Other qualities |
|---|---|---|---|---|
| Birth–6 months | Undifferentiated unpleasure | None | Relief or reduction of tension | Involves whole organism with no differentiation between self and outside object |
| 6 months–2 years | Semidifferentiated rage | Any frustrating object, animate or inanimate | Elimination of frustrating object | Self versus outside gradually achieved but still variable; presumed stage for some instances of murder, suicide, arson, etc., in children and adults |
| 1–3 years | Directed rage, tantrums, anger | Specific object, usually the mother or a sibling | Control or domination of frustrating objects; sadistic aims—hurt, torture, etc. | Talion principle ('eye for an eye') applies; control and domination of love object important, power struggles normal; gross motor discharge preferred; presumed stage for some delinquency, sadistic acts, etc. |
| 2–5 years | Modified rage and tantrums, ambivalence, jealousy, envy | Admired or feared object, usually the parents | Resolution of conflicting mixtures of love and hate, maintenance of parental love, getting even | Attempts to imitate and identify with parents, hence denial and displacement of anger is common; aggressive fantasy becomes important |

| 4–7 years | Anger, jealousy, envy | As above | As above | Internalization of rules and morals begins; fantasy and verbal expression preferred; displacement common, as onto a sibling, a scapegoat, or aggressive games |
| 6–14 years | Anger, annoyance, dislike, envy, covetousness, desire, jealousy, criticism | Peers, siblings, self | Winning, competing, assuring 'fairness', mastery of feelings | Rationality and self-control become increasingly effective; boys fight physically, girls fight verbally; substitution, sublimation, competition are typical |
| 14 years–adult | Full range of modified aggressive feelings, experienced mostly in relation to activity, work, sports | Self-attitudes become dominant | Maintenance of emotional equilibrium especially re self-esteem | Capacity for empathy with others appears, as does ability for abstract thought |

From *Conduct Disorders of Childhood and Adolescence* (Herbert, 1978), pp. 206–7, John Wiley and Sons, Inc., New York character features where early measurements – obtained at age 4 – correlate highly in boys with measurements of the same features aged 14 – possibly also because the Western culture encourages aggressive behaviour in boys. There is evidence from cross-cultural studies that contemporary Western child-rearing methods encourage tolerance for fighting and other aggressive behaviour, while traditional non-industrialized agricultural groups impose more constraints on childhood aggression (LeVine 1970).

Recent experiments have concentrated on determining how the influence of the media increases the likelihood of aggressive behaviour. The amount of time children spend in front of the television screen is astonishing: children are, according to surveys, the largest minority audience for television in Britain. In a study of 9-year-olds in an inner-city area of London (Pollak 1979) the time spent in front of television of this group is even above the average for other audiences: practically all the 139 children seen in the study (more than 95%) had watched 'telly' during the evening before their interview and the study showed that the children spent between 23 and 27 hours per week watching the screen (excluding weekends, when the time of watching still increases). This compares with the average watching time of 19 hours 12 minutes calculated as average for adults in Britain (Bugler 1976).

Almost half of the inner-city children (48.5%) looked at television whilst waiting for their mothers to come home from work. For these children, indeed, television acted as 'childminder', as suggested by Noble (1967).

The effects on behaviour of television programmes is probably vastly different according to the age of the viewers: the inner-city 9-year-olds did by no means watch only children's programmes, but often stayed up 'until it finished', thus seeing programmes with a high content of beatings, shooting and other violence intended for adult audiences. However, almost half (42.2%) of the English and West Indian children were unable to name even one of the programmes they saw the previous night. They could not remember even one, indicating that the contents must have made little impact. The *World of Disney* – certainly not a particularly violent programme – was by far the favourite. Nevertheless, there are numerous laboratory experiments carried out by social psychologists which clearly demonstrate that increased racialism and destructive behaviour follows experiences such as viewing racially prejudiced or violent films. Aggression is always increased by arousal and stimulation, and experiments indicate that anxiety, which is naturally engendered in human beings when seeing violence in life or on the television screen, diminishes with the repetition of such experiences, thus reducing the strength of the natural abhorrence which, otherwise, inhibits violence.

Researchers tend to confirm the results of Himmelweit's (1958) study, who tested 1854 children in 1950, and concluded that television violence generally does not *cause* aggressive behaviour but can precipitate it in emotionally disturbed children. Noble (1967) estimates that violence seen on the screen probably has an adverse effect on 10% of children of whom a proportion has a tendency to aggression. Himmelweit found that children were less frightened if violence on the screen was stylized and occurred in unfamiliar settings such a fairytales or Westerns, but she agrees that realistic violence, where the setting is familiar, can make viewers more aggressive and whether the victim of the violence is seen is an important factor.

Vicariously experiencing violence and vicariously participating in violent emotions does not drain off aggressive impulses and does not keep them from expression in real life (as Noble suggests). It does not in fact generally diminish the tendency to violent activity. However, according to investigations quoted by Gunter (1980, 1981) *some* children with vivid fantasies and a tendency to daydreaming may express in those daydreams their need to react in a violent fashion to provocation. Such children seem less prone to be angered and to act out in real life.

'Prosocial messages' have recently been incorporated in hugely popular American television series such as *Sesame Street* – seen by at least 8 million children every week in the early 1970s – or *Mr Roger's Neighbourhood*, destined for children, and it has been shown that the children, in fact, remember the 'messages' aimed at improving their self-images. The children (preschool and school age) were able to apply the 'prosocial' models in situations closely similar in nature to those seen on TV. However, there are no satisfactory studies to prove conclusively that these models generalize to life situations not closely similar to those situations seen on the screen, nor that the influence is more than short term, although – if used as a teaching medium – TV can help to decrease children's anxieties over dogs, dentists, etc. since the visual impact powerfully reinforces spoken teaching material.

An investigation made by Rubinstein *et al.* (1976) which assessed broadcast television programmes for their prosocial or antisocial content and the influence on children watching 'telly' found that the less TV a child watched and the more 'prosocial' his or her favourite programmes were, the more the child was likely to behave in a prosocial manner. Moreover, Gunter points out that aggressive behaviour on TV is blatant and physical, while prosocial behaviour is more subtle and inobtrusive and – as children learn better from simple, direct and active presentations – they are more likely to learn violence than prosocial messages.

In the Cambridge longitudinal study (West and Farrington 1973a) of 440 boys, seen at first aged 8–9 years, in six Primary schools and followed up to early adulthood, harsh parental attitudes were the strongest predictors of violent delinquency, and lack of parental control was the next important factor (lack of parental control was most evident in the impoverished families). Eron *et al.* (1971) carried out a study in the late 60s with all 8-year-old schoolchildren throughout Columbia County – children and parents were interviewed and filled questionnaires and sociometric methods were used. All children were judged by their peers as to the degree to which they showed tendencies to aggression in school. This study similarly came to the conclusion that aggression in school was highest in children whose parents often quarrelled with each other, were rejecting and non-nurturant. These features were conceptualized as frustrating the child and arousing his anger – establishing a state by which the probability of aggression was increased. Where the child was closely identified with the father and had internalized his rules, punishment by father was successful in reducing aggressive behaviour in school. Children *not* identified with father were highest in aggression, if father tended to punish them severely (and used physical punishment). In fact, the authors say 'anticipated punishment facilitated rather than inhibited aggressive behaviour in school'.

The treatment recommendations resulting from the team's study agree with those obtained from others. They believe firstly that to reduce the tendencies to violence aggressive models (such as violence on TV) must be made less available; secondly, that reduction of the instigation to aggression in the family (i.e. rejection, marital discord and non-nurturant behaviour) should be reduced; thirdly, that non-aggressive models should be made available; and fourthly, the consequences of aggression should be so programmed that non-aggressive behaviour is rewarded. Violent behaviour should not be followed by equally noxious negative and aggressive methods since they would lead only to imitation.

This chapter discusses the normal social development of children in the period when in addition to the influence of the home, they are submitted to powerful influences from outside: major social institutions such as schools, peer groups and mass media achieve their effects and exert intense pressures. They encourage conformity, demand impulse control and teach social skills and the manipulation of others. It is a time of testing how far what is learned in the family stands up to the challenges and scrutiny of other sources.

Groups in the middle-school years exert an immense influence. They are hierarchically structured; the members share their values. The groups' central theme is the stress on solidarity, exclusion and inclusion. This may express itself in racialism, since solidarity is based on belongingness. Intergroup rivalry may develop. Inter-racial and socially mixed schools help to mitigate the detrimental effects of this development which is, after all, part of a normal growth pattern through which children come to terms with the wider society. Social isolation, however, in the middle school years may for some individuals lead to alienation and may be experienced as a disastrous handicap.

The developmental clinician as well as teachers can help by looking into the causes of isolation. They may have to determine whether it is due to environmental factors (such as the isolated child having the 'wrong' clothes, being ashamed of their parents' behaviour, etc.) or to the child's intrinsic emotional make-up. In the last case the clinician may have to decide whether the problem is amenable to intensive treatment. Feelings of being deviant, of not fitting into the society in which one has to live, may aggravate the problems of adolescence when new social demands confront the growing child.

# Chapter 7

---

# SOCIAL ADJUSTMENT IN ADOLESCENCE

---

## (A) TIMES OF STORM AND STRESS?

Adolescence has been considered the most vulnerable and hazardous period in human development. This is how Anna Freud described it in 1937:

'Adolescents are excessively egoistic, regarding themselves as the centre of the universe and the sole object of interest and yet at no time in later life are they capable of so much self-sacrifice and devotion. They form the most passionate love relationships to break them off abruptly as they began them. On the one hand they throw themselves enthusiastically into the life of the community and, on the other hand, they have an overpowering longing for solitude. They oscillate between blind submission to some self-chosen leader and defiant rebellion against any and every authority. They are selfish and materially minded and at the same time full of lofty idealism. They are ascetic but will suddenly plunge into instinctual indulgence of the most primitive character. At times their behaviour to other people is rough and inconsiderate yet they themselves are extremely touchy. Their moods veer between light-hearted optimism and blackest pessimism.'

The description of popular, less sophisticated writers, however, is more forcefully negative: there is the image of the adolescent as egocentric, glamorizing leisure rather than work, eternally in search of kicks and excitement, considering boredom the worst of sins, etc. More scientific researches, on the other hand, generally assert that the pattern of normal adolescence is not one of volcanic eruption, but of a gradual shift towards maturity and that the pattern has not changed as fundamentally as might have been expected considering the changes within the Western society which have taken place in the last century. Rutter (1979b) said: 'The concept of parent–child alienation as a usual feature of adolescence is a myth', and 'the generation gap widely proclaimed as a source of disturbance for adolescents is a half-truth' and 'for most teenagers adolescence is not a period of either psychological disturbance or social alienation.'

King (1973) said: 'Turmoil and conflict are not necessarily the hall marks of adolescent development. Identity conflict is not common.' Rutter believes that, in fact, the generations seem to draw together more and more; certainly the gap between parents and adolescents was far wider in the period after the First World War when, at least in the middle and the upper classes, the older generation, steeped in tradition, was unable to understand the profound changes in values which had occurred at that time. He pointed out that, for instance, a close study of the Hippie culture in the 1960s showed that this movement was less one of rebellion than an attempt to implement the values of their socially conscious and politically radical parents (they tended to come from privileged families).

The picture of the rebellious, drug-taking, delinquent adolescent is based on clinical rather than normal populations. Rutter (1979b) believes that most normal adolescents still look to their parents for guidance on major decisions, while they look to peers for norms in fashion and leisure activities. The fear of restriction on their freedom by their parents, often expressed by boys, occurs only at the end of the adolescent period.

Adolescence lasted only a short time in the late 18th century when 'storm and stress' (*Sturm und Drang*) was first formulated as a feature of youthful rebelliousness and suicidal melancholy, portrayed by the young Goethe in *Die Leiden des jungen Werthers*, was followed by a wave of suicides. There existed then only a comparatively small group of students and there was no prolonged period of education for the majority, when the relatively mature youth was still dependent on the family. Physical maturity also started later in those years than it does now (menarche has advanced 4 months per decade during the last century), and puberty now begins at 10–12 years in girls and 12–14 years in boys. Young men began work long before our present school-leaving age. The adolescent culture, as we know it, is historically recent, even though the problems linked to the physiological and psychological transition from childhood to full maturity were always present.

In psychoanalytical literature the character of the so-called latency period, between 6 and 12 years of age, had been mistakenly seen as a time where sexual activities and thoughts were dormant, while sexual interests are increasing during that period, though heterosexual social activities are indeed unusual. Analytical theory assumed that puberty suddenly revived the sexual problems of early childhood and that the instinctual revival at puberty upsets the *modus vivendi* between the ego and the id. Anna Freud (1937) says that the repression of the latency period is no longer sufficient to restore emotional equilibrium and new defences have to be found to cope with the resurgence of powerful instinctual needs.

According to Rutter (1979b) it is this view of adolescence, discovered and documented by the analysts, as well as Erikson's (1968) views of adolescence as a 'psycho-social moratorium' and a time of 'identity crisis', which contributed to the view of adolescence as an overwhelmingly meaningful event. However, other factors, novel in history, contributed still more: as the period has lengthened when the young are physically mature but society has no use for them, adolescents have become an important market. Commercial interests, discovering a rich source of potential customers, have fostered the idea of adolescents as a separate group with their own culture. 'Psychosocial adolescence', Rutter (1979b) says, 'is created by society and has no necessary connection with the developmental process'. The enforced delay of productive work, the reduced importance of the extended family as a unit of social cohesion and social activity, the separation of adolescent youths into mass institutions such as school and college, and the withdrawal of any social function beyond the individualistic goal of 'self-improvement' are quoted by Coleman (1974) as factors which contribute to the separateness of the adolescent group from adult life. Society has to a certain extent sanctioned and institutionalized rebelliousness for the late adolescent years as an expected phenomenon.

Nevertheless, even if the storm and stress, the emotional turmoil said to characterize all adolescents, has been exaggerated – and probably characterizes essentially only the minority which comes to psychiatric and judicial attention – adolescence has specific features setting it apart from earlier development and imposes severe strain.

## (B) SPECIFIC SOURCES OF STRESS

The length of adolescence has advantages as well as disadvantages: the problems confronting the young do not all have to be solved at the same time. Nevertheless, the long period of dependency on the family at a time when the young have a need to free themselves psychologically from parental pressures provides countless opportunities for clashes and strains. Moreover, the adolescent has to cope with tasks and demands specific to his age. There is the developing sexual maturity, bringing anxieties about sexual competence. This includes a number of learned components and the sources of this learning are ill defined: according to a survey carried out in 1971, learning about 'facts of life' occurred (in England) in most cases at about 12 years of age and all of the interviewed children expressed dissatisfaction with the sex instruction given to them in school.

Only a few boys and even fewer girls said that they enjoyed their first heterosexual experience and two-thirds of all adolescents were disenchanted. Moreover, their knowledge of VD was scrappy. According to Kinsey *et al.* (1948) the majority of youths have severe anxieties about sex for a long time and the inhibitions, the feelings of fear, guilt and embarrassment acquired in the prepubertal period are only slowly overcome. Relative freedom of fear concerning sexuality is one of the tasks for late adolescence.

A second source of strain are the worries about *school* and *college examinations* which may decide status and earning capacity in the future. Success or failure in these tasks may seriously affect the youth's self-esteem, his concept of personal worth, increasing the uncertainty about what the future will bring. There are hormonal changes which may be the cause of emotional *mood swings*. Adolescence is a period of steep increase in the incidence of depressive illness (though it is still below adult level), while the incidence of attempted suicide is one of the most distinctive features of adolescence (since 1962 admission for parasuicide has risen tenfold for adolescent boys and fivefold for adolescent girls, and suicide comes second after accidents as the cause of death in the young). There is a fourth source of strain: the new importance of *peer relationship* and the anxiety about acceptability and popularity within the group and finally there is the risk of psychosocial disorder, delinquency and drug-taking.

## (C) JUVENILE DELINQUENCY

Juvenile delinquency is a complex issue which can be dealt with only in outline in this book. Parents may bring their teenage child to the clinician after a single incident of vandalism or stealing, but it is important to emphasize that one isolated instance is of no prognostic value. Most anti-social children do not become antisocial adults and one half of juvenile delinquents are never seen again after their first appearance in court. West recently reported on the follow-up study of children of six primary schools (seen for the first time aged 8–9 years and followed up at 21–25 years) (unpublished observations 1981); more than one quarter (136) of the 441 boys were convicted for some offences during these years. He added 'truly law-abiding' juveniles are almost deviant.

Less than one third of those convicted were recidivists and he concluded that trivial delinquency until 21 years of age is a 'self-limiting disease of youth' and an optimistic prognosis for most is justified. There remains, however, a small core of juvenile delinquents who become criminals. They almost always began their antisocial activities long before their first court appearance; they were antisocial in school, often truanting, had low intelligence scores and their antisocial behaviour was closely associated with fa-mily pathology (broken homes, large families, mental inst-ability in parents, etc.). Interestingly, in 1950, two-fifths of adolescent delinquents came from father-absent families, compared with one tenth of matched non-delinquents.

On the other hand, delinquency starting *after* adolesc-ence is not associated with these sociopathic factors. Treat-ment and judicial response to juvenile delinquency have been shown to be most difficult and least successful (see Chapter 8). It is significant that, according to a study by West and Farrington (1973b), youths with self-reported delinquency scores aged 14 were compared with respect to

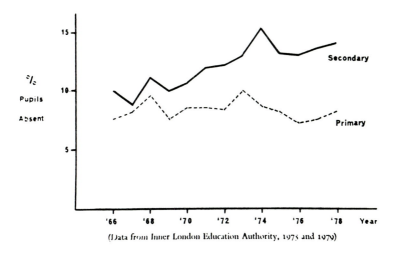

(Data from Inner London Education Authority, 1975 and 1979)

Figure 11    Trends in school absenteeism [reproduced from *Changing Youth in a Changing Society* (Rutter, M., 1979), p. 108, Nuffield Provincial Hospitals Trust, London, by kind permission]

their scores at age 18, according to whether they had received a guilty verdict in court. Those who had received a guilty verdict were more likely to be seen again, whereas the scores of those who had not appeared in court tended to fall. The reasons for the significant increase in juvenile crimes within recent years are largely obscure: increased urbanization with greater incidence of broken homes, divorces and one-parent families resulting in poor parent supervision, combined with harsh discipline in the context of unloving relationships, are probably the most damaging factors.

Moreover, the steeply increased absenteeism from school in the teenage years (Figure 11) – particularly since the raising of the school-leaving age to 16 – causes boredom to the absentee schoolboys who in gangs engage in antisocial activities. Finally, the exposure of the young to images of violence in television films and magazines – as discussed in the previous chapter – is a further influence towards destructive behaviour.

## (D) DEPRESSION AND SUICIDE

Depression, however, may be a factor in adolescent conduct disorder (Masterton 1970). 'Acting out' behaviour is now seen by many clinicians as a defence against depression. It is of utmost importance that the clinician responds to the adolescent's distress and senses the feelings of helplessness which a youth tends to hide from his parents. Depression in adolescents often presents an atypical picture and consequently the diagnosis is easily missed: while for years it was argued that depression does not occur in young people (Toolan 1971), it is now known that even young children suffer from depression.

In girls aged 8–11 years depression shows itself by bouts of weeping, loss of appetite, fears of death and schoolphobia. Later on, it may show itself in consistent ruminations, in apathy to school and family, feelings of guilt and unworthiness masked by denial, hostility or withdrawal into fantasy. Dreams of dead people are not infrequent. Restlessness, temper outbursts, experimentation with drugs in the hope of relieving feelings of estrangement are symptoms, as well as particular moodiness and self-depreciation. Suicide is rare in prepubertal children, but the incidence rises sharply in adolescence, and attempted suicide is a disorder characteristic for this period.

Although fewer adolescents than adults die from suicide, the incidence of successful and unsuccessful suicides together is above that for adults. In the Isle of Wight study, 12% of all 14–15-year-olds had suicidal thoughts. Many researchers believe that it is unjustified to describe suicidal attempts as 'not serious' or as 'blackmail', although telephone calls for help after the act are common. The underlying mood rarely differs between the successful and the failed suicides. Haim (1974) points out that the vagueness of all statistics about suicidal attempts in young people may reflect the need of society to ignore or repress the problem – it is, after all, unbearably painful to acknowledge that a great proportion of the young in our society try to escape it through death. Factors such as economic deprivation are not triggering factors in adolescents in England; the suicide rate in students is 3–6 times higher than that found outside university. Some of the 'triggers' leading to suicidal gestures are trivial: rows with girlfriends, poor school performance, etc. More important is social isolation. An estimated 30% suffer from atypical depression. But there are probably more deep-seated motivations of suicide where the trigger factors are only coincidental.

The fear of death, present since childhood, emerges in adolescence and preoccupation with the meaning of life and death is typical in this period. The idea of voluntary death as the ultimate manifestation of independence and freedom is attractive. However, there are immense reserves of energy in the normal adolescent, which prevent ideation from becoming real and it is not those who most frequently contemplate the idea of death who kill themselves. Suicides are not caused by intellectual factors. A tendency to act and to discharge impulses – in the absence of abilities to communicate feelings – though not causing suicide, leads to the use of methods which are readily available (and often inadequate to kill).

However, those who use inadequate methods, as well as the successful suicides, have often suffered feelings of uselessness before adolescence. They have had shifts of mood, felt unexplained sadness, experienced a death of a father. In some cases they have a poor paternal image – it is the father who is the link to reality – they were always socially isolated and often failed their examinations. Stengel and

Cook (1961) have drawn attention to the similarity of suicide attempts to the ancient 'ordeals' and 'rites of initiation': the need to put oneself to test, to run risks, to feel that one's worth has been proved if one has survived.

This links adolescent suicide to the incidence of accidents in youths, some of which may be unconscious or semiconscious suicidal attempts. The importance of the diagnosis of suicidal risk is immense; pointers are: an excessive tendency to act out, difficulties with verbalization, social isolation and the occurrence of events which may be experienced as irreparable loss, perhaps threatening the adolescent's self-esteem. Postponement of challenges (such as examinations) may be helpful. Availability for consultation, at times helped by medication, and an attempt by the therapists to teach the youngsters to talk and to express themselves in words, may be therapeutically helpful. (Treatment problems will be discussed in the next chapter.)

## (E) THE PROBLEM OF SEXUAL ADJUSTMENT

Biological development and emotional readiness for a heterosexual relationship do not occur at the same time and do not develop at the same pace. Even though within the last decade sexual codes have changed and openness in discussing sex is common, this does not mean that the psychosocial blocks preventing early conflict-free heterosexual relationships have been entirely removed. According to recent studies (D. and J. Offer 1971), only 10% of adolescents have had sexual intercourse before the age of 18 years and 38% before 19. On the basis of their studies of 800 boys and 400 girls, the authors conclude that emotional as well as social taboos are still very evident in adolescent behaviour. The study of a comparatively small number of sexually promiscuous girls shows the danger of too early sexual gratifications: early promiscuity cuts short the same-sex friendships, prevalent in normal teenage girls. Such friendships are necessary for socialization and are an important source of learning about social norms, to help the youth to get away from the pattern established in the nuclear family, where mother is the sole and often an unsatisfactory model for behaviour.

## (F) SEX DIFFERENCES IN SOCIAL EXPECTATIONS

Douvan and Adelson (1966) reported on interviews and test results of 1045 American boys aged 14–16 and over 2000 girls aged 12–16 (all were schoolchildren and the investigators therefore missed the lowest income groups). They also came to the conclusion that normal teenagers, far from universally rejecting parental values and rebelling against society, in fact tend to avoid conflict with parents.

Clashes over hairstyles, fashions, etc. are trivia, leaving the fundamental agreement between children and parents unaltered. The authors say, however, 'there are not one adolescent crisis but two major and clearly distinctive ones, the masculine and feminine'. Some traditionally conceived problems of adolescents, such as detachment from external authority and the dissolution of childhood object ties are not, they say, 'part of the feminine phrasing of adolescence'.

In their survey, boys have realistic fantasies of future achievements (only 15% choose 'downward mobile' jobs, jobs which are below the standard of their fathers). It is only the 'downward mobile' group which harbours feelings of hostility against authority and who reject the values of capitalist society who tend to be rebellious and withdrawn. It is this group, often sexually and psychologically immature and coming from families where hard punishment is the rule, who depict authority as arbitrary in projective tests, though they denied family conflicts to the interviewers and on questionnaires.

Most of the boys in the research were socially ambitious

and the authors say that 'the occupational issue forms the core of the masculine identity'. The boys' fantasies focus on work and achievement. They are not much coloured by dreams of glory. The boys' self-esteem depends on the success of their work and their skills. On the other hand, girls are more at home with their fantasy world. The themes that dominate their daydreams are personal attractiveness and popularity. Their self-esteem is anchored in interpersonal relations rather than in achievement. 73% of girls between 14 and 16 worry about acceptance by peers as against only 20% of boys of the same age, and over half would like to change some aspect of their physical appearance, while less than a third of boys express similar wishes.

## (G) THE FEAR OF MATURATION: OBESITY AND ANOREXIA

It is part of the need for approval, the stress on one's appearance, which manifests itself in eating disorders, a common characteristic of adolescents. Obesity, common in both young boys and girls, is a complex clinical condition, often indicating underlying emotional and social problems (Bruch 1971).

Bulimia may reflect, on the one hand, a desire to be strong and on the other hand a refusal to be attractive. It also is the cause of severe secondary social problems since the obese adolescent may be rejected by others, resulting in withdrawal from social contact and obsessive preoccupation with weight. In fact, children tend to reject those with an obesity problem. (In one sociometric study, 10–11-year-old children invariably ranked as their last choice the picture of an obese girl when required to say with whom of several they would like to be friendly.) Moreover, obesity in boys is considered to indicate lack of masculinity, which may have serious psychological consequences for the young adolescent. He may be paralysed by the fear of sexual deficiency leading to sexual dysfunction.

One third of obese children outgrow their problem, but where food stands for unfulfilled needs and is used to allay anxiety about the threatening problem of adolescence, the condition needs treatment. Bruch (1971) says that: 'To eat what one wants is considered an adult privilege and the adolescent often is rudely outspoken about refusing or demanding specific foods. In the healthy, the temporary imbalance in food intake rights itself with maturity, but the obese adolescent, according to the experiments of Schachter (1968) is not aware of his internal sensations. He does not recognize signals of hunger and satiation coming from his body and external cues such as the sight of food and its availability determine his food intake. Hunger awareness is not entirely innate, but contains an element of learning which the obese adolescent has failed to acquire.'

Obese adolescents often become classic anorectics, i.e. they either starve themselves although they are hungry, or they go on eating binges. Anorexia nervosa is five times more common in girls than in boys and more prevalent in middle-class than lower-class girls. It is a typical illness of adolescence and, like obesity, a complex condition, where emotional, personal and family problems are entangled with physiological dysfunction.

Crisp (1980) who studied a great number of anorectics, deplores the fact that the name implies loss of appetite while, on the contrary, the anorectic displays an excessive interest in food, but imposes on herself a prohibition on eating or retaining food, due to a terror of gaining weight. Crisp (1980) says that 'the primary experiential behavioural determinant of the condition is routed in adolescent concern about body shape, fatness and weight'. This is in contrast to childhood eating disorders such as the refusal of eating solids, food fads or pica which, if not due to

organic causes, are mostly due to faulty mother–child relationships. Anorectics would always eat, even hugely, if
it could be done without gaining weight, and many learn
to eat without weight gain by binging and vomiting
the ingested food, with sinister medical consequences.
30% of all 'cured' anorectics finish up with binging and
vomiting.

Anorexia, according to Crisp (1980), is always 'preceded
by a social maturational crisis which the illness serves to
resolve'. The adolescent does not feel equipped to become
a competent adult, and she is obsessed with her need to
keep her body weight below the limit where menstruation
and pubertal development are inevitable. Within the course
of the illness typical psychological and physical problems
occur, often obscuring the initial underlying obsession: the
illness arrives on the brink of adolescence and constitutes
a massive retreat from the challenge of growing up. There
is the 22-year-old girl who breaks into tears because her
doll's house has not come for Christmas. There are the
compulsive shop-lifters; at first stealing the food they dare
not keep at home through fear of eating it and going on to
steal whatever they find desirable. The girls withdraw from
social life, devote all their energy to academic pursuits (or
to cooking) and inevitably sexual commitments are impos-
sible due to their skeletal appearances (though in some
cases of continued binging and vomiting girls were promiscuous).

Anorectics are best treated in hospitals (even in those
cases where starvation or vomiting are not yet life threatening). In hospital it is not too hard to restore normal weight,
despite the fact that some reluctant anorectics use complex
ruses to prevent therapists and nurses from realizing that
food is not eaten but smuggled out of the building, hidden,
or thrown down the lavatory. However, relapses after
'cure' are common. Intense therapy is, according to Crisp
(1980) needed for a long time, to help the adolescent and

her family to accept her maturing body and eventual adult responsibility.

## (H) PROBLEMS OF PARENTING ADOLESCENTS

The handling of problematic adolescents is one of the most difficult tasks confronting parents. In despair and in fear of mishandling this period, parents bring their problems to social workers, psychiatrists and paediatric clinicians. Haim (1974) describes the parental position as the most remarkable instance of human ambivalence and says it is essential that parents should acquire insight.

They are tempted to manipulate the adolescent so that he will fulfil all his inherent potentialities. The parents try to make him all *they* would like to have achieved themselves. The child rightly resents this tendency to parental omnipotence and finds another love object. To keep the child in the family and for themselves the parents may present themselves as eternally young or they assert their authority and seniority. The adolescent, Haim says, represents to the adult both a lost paradise, their own youth, or their painful past.

Szurek (1971) draws attention to the difficulties parents experience in perceiving beneath their children's self-assertion, the tormented uncertainty, the self-doubt and anxiety about their attractiveness and abilities. The adolescent is separated from childhood by the change in his body and his cognitive maturity.

On the other hand, he is excluded from the world of adulthood for which he is not fully prepared. He may therefore turn with passionate intensity to others: there are the crushes on teachers or friends, the interminable telephone calls, the competitive emulation of outsiders' style of living, clothes and hairstyles, implying a rejection of the child's own home. This is often associated with a disdain for the ordinary rules prevailing in the parental surroundings, failure to help in chores, forgetting meal times, etc.

This is difficult for parents to tolerate. On the other hand, the adolescent is mostly so over-sensitive to criticism, because of his own uncertainty and shaky self-esteem, that any such criticism is felt as utter rejection. Moreover, parents may feel guilty and blame themselves for the adolescent's defiance; this feeling of guilt, sensed by the adolescent, again shakes his trust in the parents, which in turn contributes to his alienation from the home.

The parents may need help by the paediatrician to establish a balanced attitude to their young. They must remain firm in those demands which they see as essential, together with tolerance for temporary rebellion. They will have to realize that the quarrels about trivia, so common in this period, about musical fads, etc., must not be seen as more than symbols for the struggle towards independence. They are not really fundamental rejections of parental values in important areas. It is here where counselling may be of inestimable value for social adjustment in adolescents.

In this chapter, concerned with normal social development during the time span after school and before adulthood, I had to devote a good deal of space to deviation from normality: depression, suicidal attempts, difficulties with heterosexual adjustment, obesity and anorexia nervosa, delinquency and drug-taking are conditions typical for this age group and often continue into maturity. The high incidence of such deviance is closely linked to the particular organization of Western society. The adolescent is expected to perfect his social skills, to expand his social world and to become comfortable with heterosexual relationships, while society in some ways rejects the adolescent and has no use for his working capacity. This discrepancy leads to demoralization. The longer the twilight lasts between childhood dependency and the attainment of adult status, the more this period becomes one of irresponsibility, of emphasis on fun, and of disdain for effort.

The developmental paediatrician has no power to change the social conditions which contribute to stress in adolescents. He has no influence on the labour market, but together with teachers, social agents and parents he may be able to help the adolescent to gain insight into the fundamentally transient nature of his problem. He may advise a lessening of pressure for achievement in the years of extreme vulnerability, allowing the development of maturity to proceed at a slow pace, appropriate to the individual adolescent's needs.

# Chapter 8

## ASSESSMENT AND TREATMENT

What can be done to alleviate the plight of parents with children of deviant social development? How can the feeling to be unloved and to be unable to get along with others be relieved? And how can society be protected against the misdeeds of maladjusted and antisocial children and adolescents?

Assessment and treatment methods vary considerably according to the theoretical concepts held by therapists about the aetiology and the natural course of the various conditions. They differ still more widely according to the age of the children and the environmental circumstances in which the deviant development has arisen.

A systematic and thorough assessment of the problem and its manifestations is the first step to treatment. There are numerous tools and techniques, some of which were constructed for adults and adapted for children, some of them tailored for children directly or adapted to answer specific questions. Some of them take account of the fact that children have no words for their feelings or are reluctant to talk. Methods must be used where words are superfluous and are not an essential tool for assessment.

### (A) ASSESSMENT BY FREE PLAY

There are various play therapies combining assessment and

treatment: child therapists have toys at their disposal, grad-
uated for specific ages. In Bentovim's words (1976) 'the
therapist's understanding of children in trouble relies on
the child's tendency for unpleasant experiences to be
"played out" or "worked-over" in the mind and therefore
available for communication' in the security of the therapeutic situation. Bentovim points out that the toys are not
meant to be educational or to give the child a joyous time,
but they are meant to lend themselves in some way to
representing the child's fantasies. From the choice of the
toy, the way he plays, the therapist infers the underlying
mood: anger, anxiety, disgust, etc. The therapist may put
these moods into words for the child and make him aware
of his feelings: Do the cars *always* crash into each other
and are smashed *and* destroyed? Is the doll *always* misbe-
having and being punished? The therapist takes part in the
play, discusses what happens to the toys – symbolic repre-
sentations of the persons or objects of the child's environment. He allows the child to express hostility and anger
without the fear of being overwhelmed by disastrous consequence. He helps him to clear his confused feelings and
to distinguish between negative and positive affect, teaching him that they both may be present at the same time.

## (B) ASSESSMENT BY STANDARDIZED TOOLS

There is a more precise tool for the assessment of children's
relations to parents, siblings and the environment, which
was used by the Swansea team (Hall and Stacey 1979) to
explore the feelings of hospitalized children: the Bene-
Anthony Family Relations test. The child is given cardboard-
boxes with a figure attached to them, representing father,
mother, other relations and a Mr Nobody. They post into
these boxes typed statements stating 'He loves me best',
'Never gives me a kiss', 'Quarrels all the time,' etc. and, by
comparison with norms, the tester will know whether the

child feels rejected or particularly favoured, to whom his positive and to whom his negative feelings go, how in the child's eyes the family members feel towards him. Therapy makes use of this information.

To explore the stage children have reached in their sexual identification, the 'IT' test is used: a cardboard neuter person with numerous accessories, clothing and toys, ready to fit the neuter and turn IT into, a woman, a man, a girl or a boy, informing the therapist how the child feels about the characteristics of gender.

There are drawing tests in which the child draws a person, house and a tree and interpretation is based on indications such as the relative size of each person, whether the child has drawn a female first and how the house is arranged for the different members of the family.

Bruch (1974) uses the Draw-a-Person Test for the assessment of the severity of adolescent eating disorders. She states that a poor result in this test is a warning signal of severe maladjustment and has prognostic value.


## (C) PROJECTIVE TECHNIQUES

One such technique is the 'permissive doll play', described earlier, where children sitting in front of a doll's house play with little figures, representing themselves and members of the family, and the interpreter watches what happens: whether the child transgresses rules, and how he places himself in relations to others, etc. This test has been used to compare father-absent children with those children whose fathers live at home, and it showed that boys without fathers are less aggressive in this fantasy play than others are.

There is the children's version of the Rosenzweig Picture-Frustration Study, where people are depicted in frustrating situations and the child has to tell how the anonymous individual in each picture will act and feel (Figure 12).

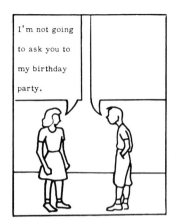 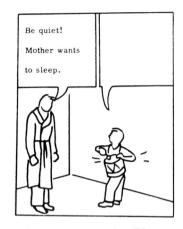

Figure 12   Two items from the Rosenzweig Picture–Frustration Study [reproduced with permission from the Children's Form, Rosenzweig Picture–Frustration Study, copyright 1975]

There are also children's versions of adult projective techniques useful only after the child can express fantasies in words. The pictures in these projective tests show children (or a puppy) in typical situations and the child's story about them will tell the sensitive listener what it is he thinks about his environment, and how he feels he is treated by the world.

Bowlby (Klagsbrun and Bowlby 1976) uses a test standardized for 5-year-old children designed to measure the extent of their anxiety in separation. It consists of a series of pictures which illustrate a variety of situations in which individuals experience loss or risk of loss. The child is then asked whether he has ever experienced an event of that kind, and if so how he felt and acted. If he has not had the experience, he is asked to imagine it and to report how he thinks he would feel. There is also the Lowenfeld World-Test, where children build a little world with toy houses, fences, children, etc., which the therapist interprets.

## (D) QUESTIONNAIRES AND SOCIOMETRY

There are innumerable questionnaires to be filled by children themselves, their parents and teachers, carefully constructed so as to elicit information about the child's observable behaviour. One of these has recently been constructed to follow up the development of children on the dimensions first measured when the Temperamental Adversity Index was established. This questionnaire measures children's attitudes to novel situations, their fastidiousness, etc. Some sociometric techniques – mostly also in the form of questionnaires – discover what children think about each other, whom they prefer to play with, whom they reject as helper in specific tasks, etc. and there is a measuring instrument of social maturity – the *Bristol Social Adjustment Guide* (Stott 1963) – which was used in the assessment of the children followed up in the National Child Development Study (Davie *et al.*, 1972). The guide contains some 250 descriptions of which the teacher underlines the one which best fits the particular child, yielding a quantitative score which can be used for statistical purposes (Figure 13).

## (E) ASSESSMENT OF ADOLESCENTS

Adolescents are being assessed by techniques used for adults: one of them, the Kelly Repertory Grid, is particularly suited to their specific identity problem. You learn by this technique what the adolescents think about 'How I am now' or 'How I would like to be' or 'The Self the other people see', etc. From the scrutiny of this test emerges a measure of the adolescent's self-esteem as well as some idea of how far he feels he is integrated in his group, how far he sees himself as isolated or different from others, etc. The Rorschach and TAT tests are also used in many of the researches on adolescents.

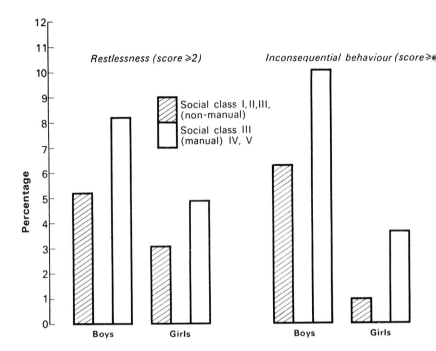

Figure 13    Bristol Social Adjustment Guide 'syndrome' scores by social class and sex [reproduced with permission from *From Birth to Seven* (Davie Butler and Goldstein, 1972), p. 150, Longman]

## (F) 'DYADIC' TREATMENT

There are two diametrically opposed methods of treating children nowadays: the 'dyadic' and the 'triadic' method. The dyadic method uses the conventional situation: the therapist confronts the child, tries to work out with him his problems and tries to understand his anxieties; he attempts to change the child's picture of the adult world by the formation of a new and confidential relationship with the therapist. Children are usually inarticulate about feelings and emotions and much of the treatment must there-

136

fore make use of non-verbal communication. Anna Freud (1968) says that it is only where the child is in true conflict that psychoanalysis is the preferred method for helping him. Where there is no conflict, therapists, in play therapy, may act as parent substitutes to understand the child's worries, assist him to find words to express his feelings or to use the toys as his vocabulary.

The child can use the toys to carry out acts on them which he cannot do in the real world – the world of the adults is too big and powerful for him, and the child therefore is confined to his fantasy world. The therapist tries to disentangle the turmoil of love and hatred, negative and positive emotions, which are the foundations of children's problems in social adjustment.


## (G) BEHAVIOUR MODIFICATION TECHNIQUES

The triadic method, fundamentally opposed to these procedures, makes use of outside persons in therapy and is based on behaviourist interpretation of childhood developmental social problems. Conduct-disordered children only rarely benefit from psychotherapy, probably because they find it hard to establish 'transference', the projection on to the therapist of their feelings about parents. They often had a thoroughly pathological relationship toward their parents and never developed a true attachment. In behaviour therapy the maladjusted behaviour is conceived as stemming from 'faulty social learning' (Herbert 1978). Treatment carried out by parents, teachers and even the child himself with the help of experts in behaviour modification focusses on the specific maladaptive behaviour, not on the child's personality or his feelings and worries. It attempts to reverse the cycle of misbehaviour, rejection and punishment, anger and repeated misdeeds. The method aims at teaching the child adaptive instead of unadaptive responses.

Isolated instances of stealing, aggressive behaviour, and hyperactivity are normally transient in children. It is only when the frequency, duration and intensity of their behaviour are so severe that the consequences for others and for the child are too damaging that treatment is needed. Treatment at units such as the Child Treatment Research Unit at the University of Leicester is performed according to learning theory principles. They assume that psychopathology can be conceptualized as inappropriate responses, acquired through learning. The unlearning of inappropriate responses is the aim of the treatment. The unit call their method 'developmental counselling' or 'behaviour casework'.

Treatment begins with a lengthy assessment aimed at precisely establishing the circumstances and frequency of the indesirable behaviour. The counsellors try to discover the consequences in the natural setting of maladaptive activities such as destruction of property, temper tantrums, compulsive eating, etc. How do parents or teachers usually react? Do they often involuntarily reinforce the undesirable behaviour by giving it attention or by allowing its reinforcement by peers?

A treatment method is mapped out in exact detail, discussed with parents and if possible in the child's presence, in order to change those circumstances which give rise to the unacceptable activity and change its consequences from reinforcing properties (i.e. tending to increase the frequency of the behaviour) to aversive properties or to replacement by other more desirable behaviour.

## (H) PRINCIPLES OF BEHAVIOURAL TREATMENT

There are some important general principles to be observed: treatment must be consistent. It must be correctly timed, so that the link between behaviour and its consequences is clear to the child. All positive assets of the child, all desirable behaviour, must be documented, praised and 'rewarded' by attention, approval and even token rewards. Physical punishment must be recognized as the least efficient consequence of undesirable behaviour. It arouses anger and feelings of frustration, and is not inducive to learning. It serves to the aggressive and impulsive child as a model to imitate aggressive, impulsive and emotional adults. Moreover, objects and people, associated with aversive stimuli, become aversive themselves.

The result of physical punishment therefore may be to escape from the punishing situation and to withdraw from the people administering it. Physical punishment may therefore have socially disruptive side effects. The general principles are: firstly, strengthening any behaviour that is incompatible with the maladjusted behaviour: secondly, the extinction of undesirable responses by changing reinforcing contingencies; thirdly, introduction in some cases of aversive consequences; and fourthly, modification or elimination of stimuli preceding the undesirable behaviour.

The literature about behaviour modification techniques is now immense, but controlled studies are still rare. Herbert (1978) lists the limitations of the procedures: improvement is not always maintained when treatment is terminated and behaviour modification does not readily transfer to situations other than the ones where intervention has taken place. Desensitization methods (for instance, as used with schoolphobic children) have also been successful, but they suffer from the limitations of most behavioural methods.

## (I) TREATMENT MEASURES IN SCHOOL

Some children constantly disrupt the discipline of the classroom, are restless, non-compliant, walk about instead of sitting down, lack concentration and tend to be 'hyperactive' (in the United States 5% of all school-age children are diagnosed as hyperactive, while only two of 2000 10- and 11-year-olds in the Isle of Wight studies (Rutter *et al.*, 1970) were so diagnosed). Teachers have been 'taught' behaviour modification techniques to enable them to get on with teaching and prevent the class suffering from the child's interruptions. Sometimes the children in the class are roped in to help in the 'treatment': they are taught to give *no* attention to unruly behaviour while praising compliance. Severely retarded children who interrupt classroom procedure are usually individually treated outside the classroom. Short periods of concentration on their tasks are rewarded and the length of this period is increased in small steps, with rewards being given at each stage of improvment. Here again, improvement is not always maintained. Moreover, teachers are used to 'negative reinforcement' methods, i.e. to admonish children for undesirable behaviour, and by this negative method they increase the attention the child receives in consequence. Teachers find it hard systematically to ignore non-compliance.

## (J) SPECIFIC TREATMENT METHODS

Behavioural methods alone are clearly inappropriate in handling severe conditions such as depression and suicidal tendencies in which diagnosis is vital and help may be urgent. The adolescent who tends to act out as a defence against depression is usually reluctant to commit himself to regular therapeutic treatment, even when he recognizes the compulsive nature of his acting out. Adolescents distrust the world of the adults and rarely come back to the therapist, once their impulse to self-destruction or their depressive moods have lifted. Those who do remain in therapy, on the other hand, may be insatiable in their demands and become hostile if the availability of the therapist is not unlimited. Nevertheless, it is essential that the adolescent should be given the opportunity to learn to express feelings and emotions in other ways than by self-destructive acts.

Group therapeutic techniques are sometimes helpful. Adolescents are particularly responsive to group pressure and many of their problems centre around peer relationships. Moreover, they often lack models for adult behaviour at a time when mothers dress like young girls. Peers in similar circumstances may help them to come to terms with reality instead of denying it. Techniques which are accepted by the young as worthwhile and not suggested by adults – such as psychodrama, the use of the expressive arts and the formation of community groups for activities – are helpful.

Varieties of residential treatment of juvenile offenders, on the other hand, according to research quoted by Rutter (1979b) 'have been fairly consistently negative in showing no overall advantage of any particular type of regime in terms of further offences'. While some specific techniques seem more successful than others inside some residential placements, generalization to situations outside the treatment centres is poor. According to Green (1977), the treatment of boys with gender confusion focusses largely on convincing the patient that he has to come to terms with reality. The child must learn to feel comfortable with his anatomical maleness. There are, however, techniques to help the 'feminine' boy to fit into the world, where masculine stereotypy is prevalent. To make him realize that he is not alone, parents may have to go out of their way to find for him companions who equally reject the pronounced masculine stereotype and who enjoy so-called feminine pursuits. Moreover, one of the main tasks of the therapist may consist in helping the boy's father to accept his son, to communicate with him and to take part in his interests and activities. The child should be helped at the same time to modify the mannerisms which single him out as 'feminine' and which draw attention to his deviancy in terms of gender sterotype.

## Family Group Therapy

This is one more of the new techniques which have not as yet proved their efficacy. It aims at analysing the communication system among family members and focusses on non-verbal communication methods. Howells (1971) says that 'its effectiveness depends on the intensity of the families' disorder'. He recommends that the therapy focus on problems of the present, and recent acute situations, while, according to him, long-standing situations are not readily solved by this method.

Some non-specific factors operate in all forms of therapy. The very encounter between child and therapist must of necessity have an impact. Features not directly attributable to the method used are often nevertheless effective, but not sufficient. The responsible therapist will in any case try to adopt his methods to the needs of the child and his particular problem. It is in early and late childhood that sometimes a treatment of the symptom only or even some manipulation of the environment is all that is needed, because the impetus of natural growth and maturation may then restore the balance. The aim of all therapy is to remove the roadblocks on the way to maturation and thus enable the child eventually to function within this social world. It is a hazardous way to travel for the child. The developmental paediatrician can help to smooth the way and spare both child and parents confusion and distress.

# REFERENCES

Ainsworth, M. D. S. (1974). Mother–infant interactions. In Connolly, K. J. and Brunner, J. S. (eds.), *The Growth of Competence*, p. 97. (London: Academic Press)

Ainsworth, M. D. S., Bell, S. M. V. and Stayton, D. J. (1971). Individual differences in stranger-situation behaviour of one-year olds. In Schaffer, H. R. (ed.), *The Origins of Human Social Relations*, pp. 7–51. (London: Academic Press)

Ainsworth, M. D. S., Bell, S. M. V. and Stayton, D. J. (1974). Infant–mother attachment and social development; socialisation as a product of reciprocal responsiveness to signals. In Richards, M. P. (ed.), *The Integration of a Child into a Social World*, p. 99. (Cambridge University Press)

Bartak, L., Rutter, M. and Cox A. (1975). A comparative study of infantile autism and specific receptive language disorder. *Br. J. Psychiatry*, **126**, 127

Bentovim, A. (1976). The role of play in psychotherapeutic work with children and their families. In Tizard, B. and Harvey, D. (eds.), *The Biology of Play*, p. 185. (London: William Heinemann Medical Books)

Bernal, J. (1974). Attachment, some problems and possibilities. In Richards, M. P. (ed.) *The Integration of a Child into a Social World*, p. 153. (Cambridge University Press)

Berney, T., Kolvin, I., Bhate, S. R., Garside, R. F., Jeans,

J. Kay, B. and Scarth, L. (1981). School phobia: A therapeutic trial with clomipramine and short term outcome. *Br. J. Psychiatry*, **138**, 110

Bettelheim, B. (1967). *The Empty Fortress*. (New York: Free Press)

Birns, B. (1977). The emergence and socialisation of sex differences in the earliest years. In Chess, S. and Thomas, A. (eds.), *Annual Progress in Child Psychiatry and Child Development*, p. 261. (New York: Brunner/Mazel)

Bowlby, J. (1946). *Forty-four Juvenile Thieves; Their Character and Home Life*. (London: Baillière, Tindall, & Cox)

Bowlby, J. (1951). *Maternal Care and Mental Health*. (Geneva: World Health Organisation)

Bowlby, J. *Attachment and Loss*, Vol. I (1969), Vol. II (1973) and Vol. III (1980). (London: Hogarth Press)

Bowlby, J. (1979). *The Making and Breaking of Affectional Bonds*. (London: Tavistock Publications)

Bowlby, J. (1980). Attachment theory: a way of conceptualizing family influences on personality development. Unpublished paper presented to the Royal College of Psychiatry, London, 21 Nov. 1980

Brazelton, T. B. (1973). Neonatal behavioural assessment scale. *Clinics in Developmental Medicine*, No. 50 (London: Heinemann)

Bronfenbrenner, U. (1979). *The Ecology of Human Development*. (Cambridge, Mass: Harvard University Press)

Brown, G. W., Harris, T. and Copeland, J. R. (1977). Depression and loss. *Br. J. Psychiatry*, **130**, 1

Bruch, H. (1971). Obesity in adolescence. In Howells, J. G. (ed.), *Modern Perspectives in Adolescent Psychiatry*, p. 254. (Edinburgh: Oliver & Boyd)

Bruch, H. (1974). *Eating Disorders*, *Obesity and Anorexia*. (London: Routledge & Kegan Paul)

Bugler, J. (1976). What's in front of the children? *The Listener*, 16 September

Burton, I. W. (1979). *The Origins of Human Competence*. (Toronto: Lexington Books)

Cairn, R. B., Green, J. A. and MacCombie, D. (1980). The dynamics of social development. In Simmel, C. (ed.), *Early Experience and Early Behaviour*, p. 79. (London: Academic Press)

Clarke, A. M. and Clarke, A. D. B. (1976). *Early Experience, Myth and Evidence*. (London: Open Books; New York: Free Press)

Coleman, J. S. (1974). *Relationships in Adolescents*. (London: Routledge & Kegan Paul)

Condon, W. (1979). Neonatal entrainment and enculturation. In Bullowa, G. M. (ed.), *Before Speech*, p. 131. (Cambridge University Press)

Crisp, A. H. (1980). *Anorexia Nervosa – Let Me Be*. (London: Academic Press)

Darwin, C. (1877). *The Expression of Emotions in Animals and Men*. (London: John Murray)

Davie, R., Butler, N. and Goldstein, H. (1972). *From Birth to Seven, a Report on the National Child Development Study*. (London: Longman)

de Chateau, P. (1980). Parent–neonate interaction and its longterm effect. In Simmel, E. (ed.), *Experience and Early Behaviour: Implications for Social Development*, p. 109. (London: Academic Press)

Dennis, W. and Najaran, P. (1957). Infant development under environmental handicap. *Psychological Monograph*, No. 436. (Washington: American Psychological Association)

Douglas, J. W. B. (1975). Early hospital admission; and later disturbance of behaviour and learning. *Dev. Med. Child. Neurol.*, **17**, 456

Douvan, J. and Adelson, J. (1966). *The Adolescent Experience*. (New York: Wiley)

Eisenberg, L. (1958). School phobia diagnosis, genesis and clinical management. *Pediatr. Clin. N. Am.*, 645–60

Erikson, E. H. (1968) *Identity – Youth and Crisis*. (New York: Faber & Faber)

Eron, L. B., Walder, L. O. and Lefkowitz, M. M. (1971). *Learning Aggression in Childhood*. (Boston, Mass: Little, Brown & Co.)

Social development

Freedman, D. A. (1965). Hereditary control of early social behaviour. In Foss, B. M. (ed.), *Determinants of Infants' Behaviour*, Vol. 3 p. 149. (London: Methuen)

Freud, A. (1937). *The Ego and the Mechanism of Defence.* (London: Hogarth Press)

Freud, Anna (1968). Indications for child analysis, and other papers. In Khan, M. M. R. (ed.). (London: Hogarth Press and the Institute for Analysis)

Freud, Anna and Dann, S. (1951). An experiment in group upbringing. In Eissler, R., Freud, A., Hartmann, H. and Kris, E. (eds.), *The Psychoanalytic Study of the Child*, vol. 6, pp. 12761. (New York: International Universities Press)

Frommer, E. A. and O'Shea, G. (1973). Antenatal identification of women liable to have problems in managing their infants. *Br. J. Psychiatry*, **123**, 149

Gesell, A. (1940). *The First Five Years of Life.* (London: Methuen)

Goodenough, F. C. (1931). *Anger in Young Children.* (Minneapolis: University of Minnesota Press)

Graham, Ph., Rutter, M. and George, S. (1975). Temperamental characteristics as predictors of behaviour disorders in children. In Chess, S. and Thomas, A. (eds.), *Annual Progress in Child Psychiatry and Child Development*, p. 16. (New York: Brunner/Mazel)

Green, R. (1977). Atypical psychosexual development. In Rutter, M. and Hersov, L. (eds.), *Child Psychiatry*, p. 788. (London: Blackwell)

Greenstein, J. M. (1966). Father characteristics and sex typing. *J. Pers. Soc. Psychol.*, **3**, 271-277

Gunter, B. (1980). The cathartic potential of television drama. *Bull. Br. Psychol. Soc.*, **33**, 448

Gunter, B. (1981). Can television teach kindness? *Bull. Br. Psychol. Soc.*, **34**, 121

Haim, A. (1974). *Adolescent Suicide.* (London: Tavistock Publications)

Hall, D. and Stacey, M. (1979). *Beyond Separation.* (London: Routledge & Kegan Paul)

Harlow, J. F. (1974). Socially isolated animal infants. In

Stone, J., Smith, T. H. and Murphy, L. (eds.), *The Competent Infant*, p. 824. (London: Tavistock Publications)

Harlow, J. F. and Suomi, S. J. (1970). Nature of love simplified. *Am. Psychol.*, **25**, 161

Hartshorne, H. and May, M. (1928). *Studies in the Nature of Characters*, Vol. I, *Studies in Deceit*. (New York: Macmillan)

Hartup, W. W. (1970). Peer interaction and social organisation. In Mussen, P. H. (ed.), *Carmichael's Manual of Child Psychology*, 3rd edn, Vol. 2, p. 361–456. (New York: Wiley)

Hartup, W. W. (1980). Peer relations and family relations – two social worlds. In Rutter, M. (ed.), *Scientific Foundations of Developmental Psychiatry*, pp. 280–292. (London: Heinemann Medical Books)

Hauser, S. L., Delong, G. R. and Rosman, N. P. (1975). Pneumographic findings in the infantile autism syndrome, a correlation with temporal lobe disease. *Brain*, **98**, 667

Herbert, M. (1978). *Conduct Disorders of Childhood and Adolescence*. (New York: Wiley)

Hersov, L. A. (1960). Refusal to go to school. *J. Child Psychol. Psychiatry*, **1**, 137

Hersov, L. A. (1977). School refusal. In Rutter, M. and Hersov, L. A. (eds.), *Child Psychiatry*, pp. 455–486. (London: Blackwell Scientific)

Himmelweit, H. (1958). *Television and the Child*. (London: Oxford University Press)

Hoffmann, M. (1970). Moral development. In Mussen, P. H. (ed.), *Carmichael's Manual of Child Psychology*, 3rd edn, Vol. 2, p. 261. (New York: Wiley)

Howells, J. (1971). Family group therapy. In Howells, J. (ed.), *Modern Perspectives in Adolescent Psychiatry*, p. 404. (Edinburgh: Oliver & Boyd)

Hunt, J. McV.(1964). Psychological basis for using pre-school enrichment as an antidote for cultural deprivation, *Merrill Palmer Quarterly*, Vol. 10, pp. 209–248. (Detroit: The Merrill–Palmer Institute)

Hutt, Corinne, (1972). *Males and Females.* (Harmondsworth: Penguin Books)

Isaacs, S. (1933). *Social Development in Young Children.* (London: Routledge & Kegan Paul)

James, W. (1890). *Principles of Psychology.* (New York: Holt, Rinehart & Winston)

Kallman, F. J. (1952). Comparative twin study on the genetic aspect of male homosexuality. *J. Nerv. Ment. Dis.*, **115**, 283

Kanner, L. (1949). Problems of nosology and psychodynamics of early childhood autism. *Am. J. Orthopsychiatry*, **19**, 416

King, S. J. (1973). Coping and growth in adolescence. In Chess, S. and Thomas, A. (eds.), *Annual Progress in Child Psychiatry and Child Development*, pp. 187–202. (New York: Brunner/Mazel)

Kinsey, A. C., Pomeroy, W. and Martic, C. E. (1948). *Sexual Behaviour in the Human Male.* (Philadelphia: Saunders)

Klagsbrun, M. and Bowlby, J. (1976). Responses to separation from parents: A clinical test for young children. *Br. J. Projective Psychol. Pers. Study*, **21**, 7

Klaus, M. H. and Kennel, J. H. (1976). *Maternal Infant Bonding.* (St Louis: Mosby)

Kohlberg, L. (1969). Stages and sequences in the cognitive-developmental approach to socialisation. In Goslin, D. A. (ed.), *Handbook of Socialisation, Theory and Research*, pp. 347–480 (Chicago: Rand McNally)

Konner, M. (1975). Infants and juveniles. In Lewis, M. and Rosenblum, L. H. (eds.), *Friendship and Peer Relations.* (New York: Wiley)

Landsdowne, R. (1981). *More in Sympathy.* (London: Tavistock)

LeVine, R. A. (1970). Crosscultural studies in child psychology. In Mussen, P. H. (ed.), *Carmichael's Manual of Child Psychology*, 3rd edn, pp. 559–612. (New York: Wiley)

McConaghy, J. M. (1979). Gender permanence and the genital basis of gender. *Child Dev.*, **50**, 1223

Masterton, J. (1970). Depression in the adolescent character disorder. In Zubin and Freeman (eds.), *The Psychopathology of Adolescence*, pp. 242–257. (New York: Grune & Stratton)

Mead, M. (1962) *A Cultural Anthropologist's Approach to Maternal Care: A Reassessment of its Effects*. (Geneva: World Health Organisation)

Mischel, W. (1970). Sex typing and socialisation. In Mussen, P. H. (ed.), *Carmichael's Manual of Child Psychology*, 3rd edn, Vol. 2, pp. 3–72. (New York: Wiley)

Money, J., Hampson. J. G. and Hampson, J. L. (1957). Imprinting and the establishment of gender role. *Arch. Neurol. Psychiatr.*, 77, 333

Moore, T. (1972). The later outcome of early care by mother and subsequent daily regimes. In Monks, F. J., Hartup, W. and de Wit, J. (eds.), *Determinants of Behavioural Development*, pp. 3–72. (New York: Academic Press)

Newman, L. E. (1977). Treatment for the parents of feminine boys. In Chess, S. and Thomas, A. (eds.), *Annual Progress in Child Psychiatry and Child Development*, pp. 230–239. (New York: Brunner/Mazel)

Newson, J. (1979). The growth of shared understanding between infant and caregiver. In Bullowa, M. (ed.), *Before Speech*, pp. 207–222. (Cambridge University Press)

Newson, J. and Newson, F. (1979). *Toys and Playthings in Development and Remediation*. (London: Allen & Unwin)

Noble, G. (1967). *Children in Front of the Small Screen*. (London: Constable)

Offer, D. and Offer, J. (1971). Four issues in the developmental psychology of adolescents. In Howells, J. (ed.), *Modern Perspectives in Adolescent Psychiatry*, p. 28. (Edinburgh: Oliver & Boyd)

Packer, M. and Rosenblatt, D. (1979). Issues in the study of social behaviour in the first week of life. In Shaffer, D. and Dunn, J. (eds.), *The First Year of Life*, p. 7. (New York: Wiley)

Piaget, J. (1955). *The Child's Construction of Reality.* (New York: Routledge & Kegan Paul)

Piaget, J. (1965). *The Moral Judgment of the Child.* (New York: Free Press)

Pollak, M. (1979). *Nine Years Old.* (Lancaster: MTP Press)

Power, M. J. Alderson, M. R., Phillipson, C. M., Schoenberg, E. and Morris, J. N. (1967). Delinquent schools? *New Society*, 1, 542

Richards, M. P. M. (1974). First steps in becoming social. In Richards, M. P. M. (ed.), *The Integration of the Child in a Social World*, p. 83. (Cambridge University Press)

Ricks, D. (1979). Making sense of experience to make sensible sounds. In Bullowa, M. (ed.), *Before Speech*, p. 245. (Cambridge University Press)

Robertson, J. and Robertson, J. (1967-72). *Young Children in Brief Separation.* (London: Tavistock Institute of Human Relations)

Robertson, J. and Robertson, J. (1971). Young children in brief separation, a fresh look. *Psychoanal. Study Child*, 26, 264-315

Robson, K. S. and Moss, H. A. (1970). Patterns and determinants of maternal attachment. *J. Pediatr.*, 77, 976

Rubin, Z. (1980). Children's friendships. In Brunner, J., Cole, M. and Lloyd, B. (eds.), *Developing Child.* (London: Open Books)

Rubinstein, E. A., Liebert, R. M., Neale, J. M. and Poulos, R. M. (1976). Assessing television's influence on children's prosocial behaviour (*Occasional Paper* 74-11). (Stony Brook, NY: Brookdale International Institute)

Rubinstein, J. (1967). Maternal attentiveness and subsequent exploratory behaviour in the infant. *Child Dev.*, 38, 1089

Rutter, M. (1976). Infantile autism and other child psychoses. In Rutter, M., and Hersov, L. (eds.), *Child Psychiatry, Modern Approaches*, pp. 717-739. (London: Blackwell Scientific Publications)

Rutter, M. (1979a). Maternal deprivation 1970-79. New findings, new concepts and approaches. *Child Dev.*, 50, 283

Rutter, M. (1979b). *Changing Youth in a Changing Society.* (London: Nuffield Provincial Hospital Trust)

Rutter, M. (1981). Social emotional consequences of day care for pre-school children. *Am. J. Orthopsychiatr.*, January 1981, pp. 4–28

Rutter, M., Maugham, P., Mortimer, J. and Orton, J. (1979). *15000 Hours.* (London: Open Books)

Rutter, M., Tizard, J. and Whitmore, K. (eds.) (1970). *Education, Health and Behaviour.* (London: Longman)

Sackett, G. (1966). Monkeys reared in isolation with pictures as visual input. Evidence for an innate releasing mechanism. *Science*, **15**, 1468

Sameroff, A. (1976). Early influences on development. Fact or fancy?. In Chess, S. and Thomas, A. (eds.), *Annual Progress in Child Psychiatry and Child Development*, pp. 3–31. (New York: Brunner/Mazel)

Schachter, S. (1968). Obesity and eating. *Science*, **161**, 751

Schaffer, H. R. (1971). *The Growth of Sociability.* (Harmondsworth: Penguin Books)

Schaffer, H. R. (1974). *Origins of Fear.* (New York: Wiley)

Schaffer, H. R. (1977). *Studies in Mother–Infant Interaction.*(London: Academic Press)

Schaffer, H. R. and Emerson, P. E. (1964). Patterns of response to physical contact in early human development. *J. Child Psychol. Psychiatry*, **5**, 1

Sears, R., Maccoby, E. E. and Levin, H. (1957). *Patterns of Childhood Rearing.* (New York: Harper & Row)

Serbin, L., Tonick, I. J. and Sternglanz, J. H. (1977). Shaping cooperative cross-sex play. *Child Dev.*, **48**, 942

Shaffer, D., Mayer-Bahlburg, H. F. L. and Stockman, C. L. J. (1980). Development of aggression. In Rutter, M. (ed.), *Scientific Foundations of Developmental Psychiatry*, p. 353. (London: Heinemann)

Spitz, R. A. (1946) with Wolf, K. M. Anaclitic depression, an inquiry into the genesis of psychiatric conditions in early childhood. In *Psychoanalytic Study of the Child*, Vol. 2, pp. 313–342. (New York: International Universities Press)

Spitz, R. A. (1950). Anxiety in infancy, a study of manifestations in the first year of life. *Int. J. Psychoanal.*, **31**, 138–43

Stayton, D. J., Hogan, R. and Ainsworth, M. D. S. (1971). Infant obedience and maternal behaviour; the origins of socialisation reconsidered. *Child Dev.*, **42**, 1057

Stengel, E. and Cook, N. G. (1961). *Attempted Suicide, its Social Significance and Effects*. (London: Oxford University Press)

Stern, D. (1977). *The First Relationship: Infant and Mother*. (London: Open Books)

Stott, A. (1963). *The Bristol Social Adjustment Guide*. (University of London Press)

Szurek, A. (1974). The needs for emotional health in adolescence. In Howells, J. G. (ed.). *Modern Perspectives in Adolescent Psychiatry*, p. 100. (Edinburgh: Oliver & Boyd)

Thomas, A., Chess, S. and Birch, H. (1968). *Temperamental and Behaviour Disorders in Children*. (New York: University Press)

Tizard, B. (1976). Effects of early institutional rearing. In Chess, S. and Thomas, A. (eds.), *Annual Progress in Child Psychiatry and Child Development*, pp. 52–68. (New York: Brunner/Mazel)

Toolan, J. (1971). Depression in adolescence. In Howells, J. G. (ed.), *Modern Perspectives in Adolescent Psychiatry*, p. 358. (Edinburgh: Oliver & Boyd)

Trevarthen, C. (1979). Communication and cooperation in early infancy. In Bullowa, M. (ed.), *Before Speech*, p. 321. (Cambridge University Press)

Tronick, E. Als, H. and Adamson, L. (1979). Structure of early face-to-face communicative interactions. In Bullowa, M. (ed.), *Before Speech*, p. 340. (Cambridge University Press)

Waldrop, F. M. and Halverson, C. (1976). Intensive and extensive peer behaviour. In Chess, S. and Thomas, A. (eds.), *Annual Progress in Child Psychiatry and Child Development*, p. 109. (New York: Brunner/Mazel)

Wallerstein, J. and Kelly, J. B. (1975). The effect of parental divorce. In Chess, S., and Thomas, A. (eds.), *Annual*

*Progress in Child Psychiatry and Child Development*, p. 520. (New York: Brunner/Mazel)

Watson, J. B. (1928). *Psychological Care of Infant and Child*. (Norton)

Weinstein, E. (1969). The development of interpersonal competence. In Goslin, D. A. (ed.), *Handbook of Socialisation Theory and Research*, p. 753. (Chicago: Rand McNally College)

West, D. J. and Farrington, D. P. (1973a). *Who becomes Delinquent?* (London: Heinemann)

West, D. J. and Farrington, D. P. (1973b). Self report of deviant behaviour: predictive and stable? *J. Crimin. Law Criminol.*, **64**, 99

Whiting, J. W. M. and Whiting, B. B. (1975). *Children of Six Cultures – a Psycho-cultural Analysis*. Cambridge, Mass.: Harvard University Press)

Isle of Wight Study (1970). In Rutter, M., Tizard, J. and Whitmore, K. (eds.), *Education, Health and Behaviour*. (London: Longman)

Wright, D. S. (1971). *The Psychology of Moral Behaviour*. (Harmondsworth: Penguin)

Yarrow, L. J., Goodwin, M. S. and Milowe, T. D. (1971). Infancy experience and cognitive and personality development at ten years. In Stone, J. Smith, T. H. and Murphy, L. (eds.), *The Competent Infant*, p. 1274. (London: Tavistock Publications)

Yarrow, L. J. and Goodwin, M. S. (1974). The immediate impact of separation: Reaction of infants to a change in mother figure. In Stone, J., Smith, T. H. and Murphy, L. (eds.), *The Competent Infant*, p. 1032. (London: Tavistock Publications)

# INDEX

*155*

# Index

# Index